TRAINING
FOOD

GET THE FUEL YOU NEED TO
ACHIEVE YOUR GOALS –
BEFORE, DURING AND AFTER EXERCISE

TRAINING FOOD

RENEE MCGREGOR

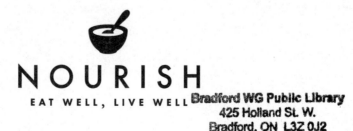

NOURISH
EAT WELL, LIVE WELL

To Andrew, Maya and Ella, for being so patient.

Training Food
Renee McGregor

First published in the UK and USA
in 2015 by Nourish, an imprint of
Watkins Media Limited
19 Cecil Court
London WC2N 4HE

enquiries@nourishbooks.com

Publisher: Grace Cheetham
Managing Editor: Rebecca Woods
Editors: Judy Barratt, Dawn Bates and
Wendy Hobson
Managing Designer: Georgina Hewitt
Designers: Briony Hartley and
Welmoet Wartena
Production: Uzma Taj

A CIP record for this book is available
from the British Library

ISBN: 978-1-84899-266-5

10 9 8 7 6 5 4 3 2 1

Typeset in Clavo
Printed in Europe

Publisher's note
While every care has been taken in
compiling the recipes for this book,
Watkins Media Limited, or any other
persons who have been involved in
working on this publication, cannot accept
responsibility for any errors or omissions,
inadvertent or not, that may be found in
the recipes or text, nor for any problems
that may arise as a result of preparing one
of these recipes. If you are pregnant or
breastfeeding or have any special dietary
requirements or medical conditions, it is
advisable to consult a medical professional
before following any of the recipes
contained in this book.

Notes on the recipes
Unless otherwise stated:
Use free-range eggs
Use medium eggs, fruit and vegetables
Use fresh ingredients, including herbs
and chillies
Use unwaxed lemons
Do not mix metric and imperial
measurements
1 tsp = 5ml 1 tbsp = 15ml 1 cup = 250ml

nourishbooks.com

CONTENTS

FOREWORD

As an athlete, I am always looking at ways I can improve my performance and this is how I was lucky enough to find Renee McGregor.

I started working with Renee back in 2010, in preparation for the European Championships in Barcelona, after striking up a friendship through our local running club. Sharing a passion for good food and running, we quickly became friends. I had been to see various other sports nutritionists over the years, but it took me no time at all to realize that she was the real deal. Renee is incredibly knowledgeable and thorough with her research; she will leave no stone unturned to get all the information before coming up with an answer. Her nutrition plans have been tailor-made to fit into my lifestyle and requirements, with practical strategies on meal ideas, snacks and race nutrition, helping to turn theory into practice. This has resulted in success for me over the marathon distance, and more recently in ultra events.

Renee helped me to understand that how I fuelled my body had a direct influence on my training and recovery. Tailoring my nutrition around my training sessions helped me take charge of my performance goals. Knowing exactly what to eat and when really helped my energy levels and accelerated my recovery time. We also worked together to create a bespoke fuelling and hydration plan for all of my major races – these ranged from road marathons in extreme heat and humidity to mountain ultras at high altitudes – again with great success. Renee's food plans are practical and realistic, which is what I was drawn to. She gives you real food choices and examples of what your meal should look like, making it easy to plan your week: invaluable for the busy lives we lead.

I can confidently say that this book is ideal for anyone looking to improve their way of eating to benefit their sport. It gives you practical, evidence-based advice on how to fuel your body to maximize your training, as well as offering lots of delicious recipes.

Holly Rush
GB Endurance Runner

INTRODUCTION

This book is for athletes of all levels, elite or recreational, young or old, experienced or new to sport. It is for those of you who want to:

>>> **Achieve your sporting goals,** whether that's improving your half-marathon time, completing your first triathlon, becoming a more powerful tennis player, or bettering your personal-best time in swimming.

>>> **Stick to a training plan** while also trying to earn a living and juggle family commitments. For example, you work late but still need to eat appropriately to get the most out of the next morning's spinning session, or you're a busy parent trying to fit your training session in before the school run.

>>> **Improve your knowledge of nutrition.** You may well know, for example, that you need to eat carbohydrate for energy and protein for recovery, but struggle to understand what that actually looks like in real food terms.

>>> **Increase your confidence** by knowing you are eating the right foods to fuel your body and maximize your training so that you can excel in your chosen sport.

When the opportunity arose to write a book about training food, with practical recipes and evidence-based nutrition, I was delighted. There is so much information about nutrition available but not all of it is backed up by science. As a registered dietitian and sports nutritionist, I have to ensure that all the advice I provide is evidence based – that is, there has been reliable research around the subject to make the claims credible and accurate.

No matter who I am working with, I see it as a collaborative journey. I first help athletes to understand the fundamentals of good nutrition and then, with practical suggestions, piece it all together to develop a nutrition plan that works for them. This is what I am offering to you here – a practical, easy-to-follow but scientific book about sports nutrition that you can tailor to your individual sport, which includes delicious, easy-to-make recipes.

HOW TO USE THIS BOOK

The reason I enjoy my job so much is because every day is different and I work with athletes of all levels and disciplines. My job is to make the science accessible. Through researching all the latest studies, and interpreting them into practical application, I produce recipes and nutrition plans that work for all lifestyles and budgets. I have used the same step-by-step approach in this book.

Chapter 1 is a practical guide of what to eat, when to eat and how much to eat. We also look at how your body metabolizes the food you eat into fuel, and how it can adapt to provide fuel for different levels of training intensity.

Chapter 2 goes into more detail about training and how making the right nutritional choices around training sessions of different intensities will benefit you. This section also includes sample menu plans, using the recipes from the book to demonstrate practically how to make appropriate choices.

Chapter 3 tailors nutrition to your chosen sport, looking at the different fuelling requirements for different events/distances. Again I have tried to make this as practical and applicable as possible by using case studies of clients I have worked with.

Chapter 4 highlights the importance of maintaining the well-oiled machine we call our body. Often individuals ignore niggles, going into denial that anything is wrong, and this leads to further complications. This chapter ensures you go through a mental checklist before you embark on training or competition in order to avoid any long-term injury and explains how nutrition can be used in injury prevention and recovery.

Throughout the book there are also 'info boxes' and 'fact boxes', as well as quick tips, which help to make the book fun and practical, while still delivering up-to-date and evidence-based sports nutrition.

MY JOURNEY

Nutrition – and sports nutrition in particular – is my passion. It was an interest of mine from a young age and led to me becoming a registered dietitian. After working for the NHS for 10 years, mainly in paediatric nutrition, I felt it was time for a change.

I have always been an active and sporty person, and had completed challenges such as the London to Brighton Bike Ride before having children. To combine my favourite pastime with my work, I studied to be a dietitian and sports nutritionist. With the help of my amazing and extremely supportive husband I also launched my own freelance business and brand, Eat Well, Feel Fab. Ultimately this is what I had always wanted – to help people to eat well, without fads or deprivation, and feel fab for the rest of their lives.

I had started running with Team Bath Athletics Club and through this I had a place in the London Marathon. I trained hard and put my sports nutrition into full use. I was a perfect case study – a busy working mum attempting her first marathon! Race day arrived and it was an incredible experience. I finished in 3 hours, 17 minutes, much faster than my goal of 3 hours 30 minutes! Since then I have continued to be my own guinea pig, trying out nutritional theories and strategies. Last year I completed my first ultra-marathon (Classic Quarter, 44 miles on the Cornish coastal path) with a top 10 female finish, followed by the highlight of my running career to date, a 7-day multi-stage race in Nepal, climbing up to 5,162m/16,935ft of altitude (Manaslu Mountain Trail Race).

At Team Bath AC we are very privileged to be coached by Martin Rush, Head of Endurance at England Athletics. He is married to Holly Rush, GB marathon runner and ultra-runner. Holly and I have become good friends and work together; I provide her with nutritional support around all her key races and she coaches me – it's a great set-up.

I became a sports nutritionist at Bath University in the run-up to the London Olympic Games, working with the GB Rhythmic Gymnastics squad, the GB Beach Volleyball team and with individual athletes. It was an exciting but challenging time, with each sport needing a different approach relating to their ages, their experience and also the demands of their training.

So it is drawing from my professional experiences as a nutritionist and personal experiences as an endurance and newly converted ultra-runner that I have written this book. I hope it helps you to achieve all your sporting goals.

CHAPTER 1:
FUELLING BASICS

FROM NOVICE TO OLYMPIAN

There is so much hype around sports nutrition these days; the science is evolving, with an increasing number of studies proving that nutrition plays an important part in performance gains. This chapter will help you to understand why correct fuelling around your training is important to achieve your goals and optimize your performance. Whether you are new to a sport, a young athlete with energy and growth demands, or a regular on the marathon circuit, getting to grips with the basics of sports nutrition can make all the difference to your results.

You will probably have some idea of the basics of good nutrition – for example, eat carbohydrate for energy, protein for repair, fat for absorption of important nutrients, and vitamins and minerals for a healthy immune system. In this chapter we will look at these factors in more detail and I will explain how the quality of these nutrients, and when you consume them, plays a fundamental role in sports nutrition. I will also explain how fuelling right will:

>>> Encourage enhanced recovery

>>> Optimize hydration

>>> Help you to achieve and maintain an ideal body weight

>>> Reduce the risk of illness and injury

Some days I work with elite, national-level athletes, other days I spend with juniors within talent development squads. Sometimes I work with the members of a football academy, and still other times I spend with recreational athletes – for example, those who do sport as a hobby but who often have a goal in mind, such as a marathon or an Ironman event. No matter who I'm working with, the journey is a collaborative one that begins with the fundamental principles of good nutrition. In fact, these principles are applicable to us all, regardless of whether or not we intend to become athletes. What is certain is that whether you're a novice or an Olympian, you need to begin with a strong nutritional foundation that will enable the more detailed nutritional plans to work their proper magic. This will make you stronger, fitter and more able to meet your performance goals.

BEFORE YOU READ ON...

When working with sports nutrition it is normal to calculate the nutritional requirements for each macronutrient to ensure that training fuel demands are being met. These are converted based on your weight in kilograms, so throughout the book I will be referring to grams of nutrients per kilogram of your body weight, or as you will see it displayed: 'g/kg BW'. Therefore, a great starting point would be to calculate your weight in kilograms. Most home scales will have conversions. Using metric values ensures greater accuracy.

THE SPECIFICS OF SPORTS NUTRITION

The main difference between healthy eating and sports nutrition is the attention to detail and the fine-tuning of nutrient delivery. In healthy eating, the ultimate goal is to promote long-term good health and fend off increased risks of disease, while maintaining a balance so that food is still enjoyable. In comparison, sports nutrition, although still based on healthy eating guidelines to an extent, is performance driven. It is about getting the best out of your training, whether that's running for 45 minutes three times a week or training to compete in an Ironman event. Making the right nutrition choices to suit not only your specific sport but the intensity of that activity within your given training session will ensure that you have:

1 > Put the right amount and type of fuel into your body to meet the demands of your session, allowing you to perform to your best ability

2 > Made the correct choices after your training session, which will allow your body to adapt to your training and make it stronger within your chosen sport

We will go into more detail about this when we discuss different intensity levels of training in Chapter 2 and individual sports in Chapter 3.

The key to good sports nutrition is preparation and organization; fundamentally, to achieve your goal you need to tailor your nutrition to the exact training session. It's not just about energy in and energy out. I have lost count of the number of athletes who think they can get away with eating poor nutrient-dense foods just because of the amount of training they do. They may well maintain their weight and have the energy to train but what they don't see are the adaptations (see page 98) that they should. So what should they see? To a degree it will depend on the chosen sport but some general gains should be:

>>> Increases in strength and lean muscle mass

>>> Improvement in performance within their chosen sport

>>> Good consistency between training sessions so that each one can be conducted to the best of their ability

>>> Good sleep patterns, good mood and high energy levels

By just meeting energy demands, you may be able to carry out all your training but you may not see any actual improvements in your day-to-day training and overall performance.

TRAINING NUTRITION

So what types of food should you eat before a training session? Remember training is the stimulus that sends messages to your muscles to work at a specific level. In order for this stimulus to work effectively, you will need to feed it appropriately. What you feed your body before training will very much depend on what the session is and its intensity.

Like most people you probably eat carbohydrate before you exercise, to give you energy. However, do you ever stop to think about how much carbohydrate you really need, for example, to go for a 45-minute run? Would this choice be different if you were going out to run 45 minutes hard or if you were just going for a bit of a plod as a social run with some friends? The reality is that you would need a lot less carbohydrate, in fact probably none, if you were just going for a plod but your body would struggle to maintain a high intensity of exercise for 45 minutes of hard running, without carbohydrate.

Carbohydrate is stored within our muscles and liver as glycogen (see page 18) and when our body signals that it needs energy, for example during exercise, it will convert this glycogen into glucose and transport it to the working muscle to ensure that the level of activity can be maintained. Although your body could get energy from fat stores, the subsequent processes to convert fat to glucose take too long and so it would not support high-intensity exercise. This is why it is so important that you fuel your body with carbohydrate prior to a hard training session.

So what happens if, for example, you have a bowl of porridge/oatmeal and then head out for a slow social plod with friends? Your body will still use the carbohydrate provided by the porridge/oatmeal as it is still the most available source of fuel. What is so bad about that, you might ask? Well nothing really, unless you want to lose some body fat or you want to become fat adapted (see page 84).

For you to use fat as fuel, you will need to work at a moderate to low intensity (we will be discussing intensity in much more detail in Chapter 2). This is because this level of activity is slow enough to allow your body time to provide the energy it needs from fat stores. So if you have a few pounds to shift or are trying to become a bit leaner, this type of training session can be useful and as long as you do it in a fasted state or ensure that your last meal did not contain carbohydrate, this is what will happen.

Some of my athletes, particularly endurance athletes, like to become 'fat adapted' – this means that their body becomes more efficient at using fat as fuel and so can help 'spare' glycogen stores in long endurance events that last longer than two hours such as the marathon, Ironman or cycling sportive. So when you think about training nutrition, the main questions you need to ask yourself are:

1 > What type of session is this going to be? High, medium or low intensity?

2 > How long is this training session going to be?

Answering these questions will help you to choose the correct fuel and the correct portion size.

CARBOHYDRATE

Most people who partake in sport will be aware of the need to consume carbohydrate as fuel for training sessions. Indeed when you look at health promotion tools such as 'the Eat Well Plate' or 'the Food Pyramid', the carbohydrate component makes up a large proportion. But do we always get the balance right? In order to answer this, we need to know the difference in the types of carbohydrate as some are more desirable than others!

In general terms, your carbohydrate requirement will depend on your activity level; it is the key fuel source for exercise as it is broken down into glucose and utilized by the body to provide energy. Carbohydrate is stored as glycogen within the liver and muscles. It is this source within the muscle that is the most readily available energy for working muscle, releasing energy more quickly than other sources. However, this storage facility is limited. If the muscles are inadequately fuelled, it will lead to fatigue, poor performance and potentially lower your immunity, putting you at greater risk of illness.

So if you are doing any sport, it is really important to plan your carbohydrate intake around training sessions; the amount you require will be dependent on the frequency, duration and intensity of your training. So on days when you have a high-intensity training session, you will need more carbohydrate and on rest days or lower-intensity days you will need less. This is summarized in the table opposite and is addressed in more detail in Chapter 2.

To help you meet your needs, it is important to understand the difference in the types of carbohydrate that are available. Over the years, carbohydrates have been classified in many different ways; the most common types are simple and complex, but you may also be familiar with high GI (glycaemic index) and low GI. The glycaemic index (GI) is a ranking of carbohydrate-containing foods based on the overall effect on blood glucose levels. Slowly absorbed foods have a low GI rating, while foods that are more quickly absorbed have a higher rating. Most recently, sports nutritionists have started to use the terms 'nutrient dense', 'nutrient poor' or 'high fat' types of carbohydrate. Nutrient-dense carbohydrates are food options that provide carbohydrate as well as other nutrients; examples include bread, fruit and dairy. Nutrient-poor carbohydrates provide carbohydrate but no other useful nutrients; some examples include energy drinks and sugar. High-fat options provide carbohydrate but also a high percentage of fat, and these foods should be kept to a minimum; examples include chocolate and pastries. These are summarized in the table below:

Category	Description	Examples	Use for athletes
Nutrient-dense carbohydrate	Foods and fluids that are rich sources of other nutrients, including protein, vitamins, minerals, fibre and antioxidants, in addition to carbohydrate.	Breads, cereals and wholegrains (eg oats, pasta, rice), fruit, starchy vegetables (eg potato, butternut squash), legumes (eg lentils, beans, peas and peanuts); low-fat dairy products (eg milk, yogurt).	Everyday food that should form the basis of an athlete's diet. Helps to meet other nutrient targets, such as good fats, protein, vitamins and minerals.
Nutrient-poor carbohydrate	Foods and fluids that contain carbohydrate but minimal or no other nutrients.	All sugars (eg dextrose, sucrose, agave nectar, honey, molasses etc); soft drinks, energy drinks, lollies, carbohydrate gels, sports drinks and cordials, any type of white bread.	Shouldn't be a major part of the everyday diet but may provide a compact carbohydrate source around training.
High-fat carbohydrate	Foods that contain carbohydrate but are high in fat.	Pastries, cakes, chips, crisps and chocolate.	Occasional foods that are best not consumed around training sessions.

TABLE 1.1 Types of carbohydrate

It is difficult to quantify what percentage of your overall diet should be formed of carbohydrate, which is why no matter who I work with, a recreational or an elite athlete, I use the guidelines in the table below. However, be aware that these are ball-park figures and will vary from individual to individual. Additionally there is a gender difference: women in general utilize a much lower amount of carbohydrate. For example, if a man and a woman sit at a desk working all day, the man will be utilizing a much higher ratio of carbohydrate for energy than the woman, who will use more fat for energy. For this reason female requirements tend to be around 10–15 percent lower than those stated here.

Exercise intensity	Situation	Carbohydrate targets for men	Carbohydrate targets for women
Light	Low-intensity or skill-based activities, such as archery, shooting and Pilates (or exercising fewer than three times per week)	3–5g per kg BW	2–4g per kg BW
Moderate	Moderate exercise programme (around 1 hour per day)	5–7g per kg BW	3–5g per kg BW
High	Endurance programme (ie moderate-to-high intensity exercise of 1–3 hours per day)	6–10g per kg BW	5–7g per kg BW
Very high	Extreme commitment (ie moderate-to-high intensity exercise of 4–5 hours per day)	8–12g per kg BW	8g per kg BW

TABLE 1.2 Carbohydrate intake requirements for different training intensities

So for most moderately active 60kg/132lb adults, who like to go for a 30–45-minute run at an easy pace three times per week, this works out to be 3 x 60g = 180g of carbohydrate a day. I recommend that this requirement is solely made up from the nutrient-dense list of foods (see Table 1.1, page 19). Even within this group, certain foods will be better as they will make your carbohydrate go further, so for example 100g/3½oz rolled oats provides 60g of carbohydrate but 100g/3½oz of butternut squash only provides 20g of carbohydrate, so you would need to eat 300g/10½oz of butternut squash to provide 60g. Here are some other examples:

>>> 100g/3½oz wholemeal bread will provide 60g of carbohydrate

>>> 100g/3½oz dry-weight pasta will provide 75g of carbohydrate

>>> 100g/3½oz beetroot/beets will provide 20g of carbohydrate

>>> 100g/3½oz mango will provide 20g of carbohydrate

>>> 1 banana will provide 25g of carbohydrate

>>> 400g/14oz drained can of chickpeas will provide 39g of carbohydrate

So by using more of the vegetables, fruit and legumes as your carbohydrate source, your allowance will go a lot further.

In one of my favourite examples of different types of carbohydrates, I compare jelly babies to sweet potatoes. Ten jelly babies provide 60g of carbohydrate. But a 300g/10oz (medium) sweet potato or six large carrots provides the same. It is obvious which option will be the more filling. This example also demonstrates how easy it is to over-consume simple carbohydrates – most people could polish off a big 190g/7oz bag of jelly babies, which would provide in the region of 152g of carbohydrate but could they consume the equivalent in sweet potatoes or carrots in one sitting?

Having said that, in certain training situations, jelly babies may be the preferred fuel. For example, you might be training for a triathlon and doing a BRICK session (bike and then straight into a run), which is going to last over 90 minutes. By fuelling up with nutrient-dense carbohydrates, such as pasta, bagels or oats, you will have built up good glycogen stores. However, these stores tend to only last between 60–90 minutes, depending on the intensity at which you train. So you will find it useful to 'top up' your stores by choosing foods from the nutrient-poor group. This is where foods such as jelly babies, dried fruits, energy drinks, jam sandwiches made with white bread or energy gels can be very useful. We will look at this in more detail in Chapter 3. Immediately after your training session is over, you will need to replenish your stores and this is the ideal time to consume something like flavoured milk, which is high in carbohydrate.

So remember, as athletes, it is important to consume carbohydrate to help fuel your training sessions. However, it is essential to choose the *right* type, at the *right* time in the *right* portion. We will look at this in more detail later on in this chapter.

FACT OR FICTION?

Does carbohydrate cause weight gain?

In recent years, there have been many mixed and confusing messages about carbohydrate, with many people believing that it is the root cause of weight gain in the Western world. But how can this really be possible when 1g of pure carbohydrate only yields 3.87 calories?

In simplistic terms, carbohydrate is the fuel our body finds easiest to use. So if it is available, your body will choose carbohydrate as its fuel source whether this is for a high-intensity training session, an hour of housework or sitting in front of a computer all day. Once this carbohydrate fuel has run out, your body will look to your fat stores to continue to provide this energy.

The confusion occurs if you consume more calories than your body needs as any excess will be stored as fat, whether this excess comes from carbohydrate, protein or fat sources. It is quite easy to over-consume carbohydrates, especially if they come in the form of non-nutrient dense varieties such as drinks and sweets, but also when combined with fat in the case of pastries or pies. Although fat has a higher yield of calories per gram of food, in general foods that contain a high percentage of fat such as cheese, certain meats, oily fish and olive oil tend to keep you fuller for longer. Fat has a slow transit time in the gut, so it slows down the absorption of food from the gut during digestion. Protein has a similar energy yield to carbohydrate per gram of food but foods high in protein, such as chicken, fat-free Greek yogurt and white fish, are more difficult to break down by the body so leave you feeling full for longer. This is the real reason why diets such as Atkins and Paleo are successful for weight loss. The Atkins Diet was devised by Robert Atkins and is predominantly a low-carbohydrate diet, promoting the intake of high fat and protein foods, including cream, butter and meat. The Paleo Diet allows certain carbohydrate foods such as sweet potato and potato but restricts the intake of wholegrains, dairy and sugar. So predominantly the diet is made up of high-protein meat and fish with vegetables.

When you remove food groups from any diet you are also restricting overall energy intake, especially if these foods are difficult to replace in a new diet. For example, a typical meal prior to embarking on the Atkins Diet might be a piece of chicken, a jacket potato and steamed vegetables. However, on Atkins you would only eat the chicken and vegetables so without even trying you have removed up to 200 calories from your daily intake. This example has little to do with avoiding carbohydrates but the overall calorie restriction. This was demonstrated in a study a few years ago where individuals were put on a diet of 1,500 calories. Half were given their calorie intake via cream cakes and the other half a balanced diet including some complex carbohydrate, protein and fat. Both groups lost weight in similar amounts but the cream-cake group felt more lethargic, dissatisfied and had severe sugar cravings.

This said, in athletes where energy restriction is necessary to lose weight the key is not to lose muscle mass as this will have a negative effect on strength and performance. In these cases increasing protein to above normal amounts is a beneficial way of helping to keep an athlete full, as protein has a high satiety value; it prevents the breakdown of muscle for fuel, therefore preserving lean muscle mass which in turn prevents a decrease in metabolic rate, often associated with low energy diets. However, such a diet should always be supervised by a qualified practitioner in order to prevent injury or illness. I would never remove carbohydrate – I would reduce it and be clever with its usage by including it at key training sessions to ensure energy availability and also to prevent sugar cravings.

PROTEIN

Proteins are often called the building blocks of the body. Protein consists of combinations of structures called amino acids. There are 20 amino acids and these combine in various sequences to make muscles, bones, tendons, skin, hair and other tissues. They serve other functions as well, including transporting nutrients and producing enzymes.

Eight of these amino acids are essential and must come from your diet. They are found as a complete source in animal-protein food such as dairy, meat, fish and eggs. They are found in an incomplete source in plant-based proteins; that is, they will be lacking in one or more of the essential amino acids. Examples include vegetables, grains, nuts and legumes. If, however, these are combined in the correct way you can make a whole source of protein. Some good combinations include baked beans on toast; rice and dhal; and wholegrain bagel with peanut butter. (See also pages 47–51 for information on vegetarian and vegan diets.)

In general terms, most moderately active adults, so those of you who walk the dog daily or stroll down to the shops and take one exercise class a week, will meet your protein requirements without any problems. The suggested amount is around 0.8–1g/kg BW per day, with women needing the lower end and men the upper of this range.

Think about your daily intake of food: chances are you will have had milk on your breakfast cereal, maybe meat, fish or egg at lunchtime and most likely the same again for dinner. It's also important to highlight here how small a portion you need to get a decent amount of protein.

Let's take a 57kg/125lb woman: based on the calculation 0.8g/kg BW per day, her daily protein requirement will be 46g/1½oz of protein. The following food portions provide 15g of protein:

>>> **2 large eggs**

>>> **75g/2½oz portion of chicken**

>>> **75g/2½oz portion of salmon**

>>> **150g/5oz pot of low-fat Greek yogurt**

>>> **400ml/14fl oz of milk**

By choosing just three of the above choices, she will have met her daily protein requirement.

Things are slightly different when you are working with an athlete. Athletes need protein primarily as a response to exercise rather than as a fuel source. Protein has been a huge area of research for many years, with the most recent findings demonstrating how important protein is in the recovery phase. During all exercise, including endurance sports such as running and cycling; team or power sports such as netball, football, tennis or resistance training (using weights); an increase in the breakdown of protein in the muscle has been shown. By ensuring good protein choices throughout the day, you will help to counteract this. Exercise acts as a stimulus for your muscles; it develops the muscles so that they work optimally in your chosen sport.

Let's take football as an example: a specific training session may involve doing repeated sprints to prepare your muscles for a match-day scenario, where a high proportion of your game is made up of sprinting. By ensuring good protein choices around your training, your body will promote muscle growth and repair to support this training session and encourage your muscles to adapt for when you are playing a football match. We will go into more detail about this in Chapter 3.

So how much protein does an athlete actually need? Some recommendations are based on g/kg BW a day. However, just like with carbohydrate, where you need to alter the amount you consume depending on your level of training, there is a similar approach with protein. As I have already mentioned, one of the key roles of protein for athletes is to stay in a positive protein balance (so there is more protein available than will be broken down during training), with a good supply of amino acids available that the body can draw from to prevent a breakdown (catabolism) of the muscle.

The latest guidelines recommend something called protein pulsing, where protein is consumed more frequently throughout the day

Tip
Contrary to popular belief, protein is just as important a component for endurance athletes as it is for power/speed athletes: it is vital for repair and recovery of muscles.

rather than as a large amount straight after exercise (you may have seen those pictures of athletes, particularly strength athletes, tucking into plates of chicken and eggs after training). The recommendations are that an athlete should consume 0.25g/kg BW 3–6 times a day. From a practical point of view this all might sound quite daunting but if you weigh 80kg/176lb this will translate as 0.25g x 80kg = 20g of protein at each sitting. The number of these protein portions will depend on the type and frequency of exercise but also on overall goals. For example:

>>> Do you want your muscles to get bigger (muscle hypertrophy)?

>>> Do you want to increase muscle strength so that it can power your chosen sport more efficiently and effectively?

>>> Do you have body composition goals (see page 58)?

>>> Are you a young athlete going through an active growth phase (see page 28)?

A 20g portion of protein would look like this:

>>> 3 large eggs

>>> 75g/2½oz (half a 150g/5oz can) tuna

>>> 100g/3½oz salmon fillet

>>> 130g/4½oz cod fillet

>>> 130g/4½oz mackerel fillet

>>> 85g/3oz halibut fillet

>>> 100g/3½oz pilchards in brine

>>> 175g/6oz peeled prawns/shrimp

>>> 200g/7oz tofu

>>> 80g/2¾oz portion of pork loin

>>> 4 pork sausages

>>> 600ml/21fl oz skimmed milk

>>> 200g/7oz cottage cheese

>>> 60g/2oz nuts – any unsalted

>>> 70g/2$\frac{1}{4}$oz crunchy peanut butter/almond butter

>>> 1 x 240g/8$\frac{1}{2}$oz (drained weight) can chickpeas/kidney beans

>>> 1 x 400g/14oz can baked beans in tomato sauce

>>> 100g/3$\frac{1}{2}$oz dry-weight lentils

>>> 100g/3$\frac{1}{2}$oz fillet chicken

>>> 60g/2oz Cheddar/feta/mozzarella

>>> 57g/2oz skimmed milk powder

>>> 25g whey powder

Eating any more than this figure of 0.25g/kg BW will have no extra advantage – it will not mean that your muscles will grow bigger quicker! The only time I will encourage a slightly higher figure of 0.30g/kg BW is if I am working with an athlete who weighs more than 80kg/176lb.

Additionally it is important to always ensure that one of these protein pulses comes immediately after exercise as a recovery choice but we will look at this in more detail on page 51 when we discuss recovery nutrition.

THE YOUNG ATHLETE

Like adults, young athletes need to fuel their bodies to reach optimum performance. But, unlike an adult, the body of a young athlete is still growing and changing, meaning that the nutritional demands on it are, in some respects, even greater. Many young athletes 'find' their sport just as they reach adolescence – you may even have bought this book because you are a teenager who is just about to start training for competitive sport (or are a parent who has a teenager doing so). If so, that's great because you have just taken the first step to ensuring that you fuel your body in the right way to be the best you can be during this important time of transition into adulthood.

Without adequate nutritional intake and energy stores, a young body can stop developing in the right way. This can mean slowing down the rate of growth of your bones (meaning among other things that you might not grow as tall as you could), as well as having low body fat and low weight (these aren't good things, by the way – see pages 58–60 to understand why), and for girls it can also mean delaying the start of their periods.

The consequences of inadequate energy are particularly severe for adolescent athletes. It is a rapid time for development and growth, particularly bones, which are developing in size and density. A restricted diet means a lower intake of essential nutrients such as calcium. This combined with the fact that overall energy availability is low means that your body needs to prioritize providing energy to live, move and breathe over reproduction, resulting in a reduced amount of sex hormones circulating in your body. These three factors result in your bones not strengthening properly, making you more susceptible to stress fractures in future years. However, all is not lost, because numerous studies show that, although it can take several years, taking positive steps with your nutrition so that you normalize your energy levels can reverse any negative impact on your body so far. Though, of course, it's better to get it right from the start! In most cases, when your nutritional intake meets your training needs, your body composition (see page 58) will follow suit.

If you are a young athlete, your energy demands are significantly greater than someone who is undertaking the same amount of exercise but who lives a sedentary lifestyle. This is partly because your body is growing and needs energy to do so, but also because you are likely to be far more generally active than someone who has a desk job during the day. Think of the times you have to climb the stairs at school, or the amount of curricular and extra-curricular sports you do in addition to your specific training schedule. It is important that the need to increase total energy intake is not seen as an excuse to fill up on energy-dense, nutrient-poor foods, such as takeaways and junk food.

First and foremost, eating and drinking must be a priority! Three main meals with snacks in between should be the aim – it's easier to eat more often than it is to eat more in one sitting. Try to plan ahead so that you always have access to suitable food and drinks when you need them most. I encourage my junior athletes to top up their kit-bag essentials. Foods such as dried fruit and nuts, fruit breads, sweet and savoury oatcakes are all good pre-training options; pots of milk puddings such as custard or rice pudding and long-life flavoured milks are suitable recovery foods. For training sessions that last longer than an hour, it may also be necessary to top up energy levels with foods such as bananas, dried fruit, jelly babies (see page 21) or diluted fruit juice (see page 37). For those of you with small appetites that struggle to eat before and after training, energy-dense drinks are a great 'top up' snack. Good choices include fruit smoothies and milkshakes (see the recipe section for some great ideas). These also help address your hydration needs; studies have shown that a 2 percent level of dehydration can affect performance and concentration by up to 10 percent. In a 50kg/110lb athlete this looks like 1kg/2lb loss in weight and means you have actually lost 1 litre/35fl oz of fluid. All this advice is remarkably similar to the advice I give adults – and that's the key. If you can follow the advice given throughout the book, including the advice for your particular training schedule and sport, you will be on the road to optimizing not only your performance, but your growth and lifelong health, too.

●●

FAT

Contrary to popular belief, not all fat is bad for you! In fact, it is vital that everyone eats some fat to help absorb fat-soluble vitamins A, D, E and K and to provide essential fatty acids that the body cannot make. These nutrients have important roles to play within the body. However, eating too much of a particular kind of fat – saturated fat – can raise your cholesterol, which increases the risk of heart disease. Saturated fat is the kind of fat found in butter and lard, pies, cakes and biscuits/cookies, fatty cuts of meat, sausages and bacon, cheese and cream. It also encompasses trans fat, which is often found in processed foods. It's important to cut down on this type of fat and choose foods that contain unsaturated fat (see below). It is also important to remember that eating too much fat leads to weight gain, as foods high in fat are high in energy too. For example, 1g of fat provides 9 calories in comparison to 1g carbohydrate, which provides 3.87 calories and 1g protein, which provides 4 calories. Being overweight will also increase your risk of getting certain clinical conditions such as type 2 diabetes.

Most of us eat too much saturated fat – about 20 percent more than the recommended maximum amount.

>>> **The average man should eat no more than 30g of saturated fat a day**

>>> **The average woman should eat no more than 20g of saturated fat a day**

To put this into context, by having butter on two pieces of toast, cheese as a sandwich filling and a bar of chocolate, you can clock up around 35g/1¼oz of saturated fat.

We should aim to eat more 'good' fats or unsaturated fats. These include:

>>> **Oily fish, such as salmon, sardines and mackerel, which are an exceptionally good source of omega-3 fatty acids**

>>> **Nuts and seeds, including their oils and butters**

>>> **Sunflower, rapeseed/canola and olive oils**

>>> **Avocados**

When I work with athletes, I like to encourage them to use these good fats as much as possible in their diets over saturated varieties. However, it is important to point out that these good fats still have a high-energy value and should be eaten with that in mind.

I generally recommend you take on around 1g/kg BW fat in total a day and that the majority of this comes from good fats. So for a 60kg/132lb athlete this will be 60g. I give all my athletes a list similar to the one opposite and encourage them to choose servings off the list to make up their daily requirements:

>>> 25g of nut butter (14g of fat)

>>> 100g/3½ oz avocado (15g of fat)

>>> 20ml of rapeseed/canola oil (18g of fat)

>>> 25g sunflower seeds (13g of fat)

>>> 1 mackerel fillet (16g of fat)

So for a 60kg/132lb athlete this would be two slices of toast with 25g peanut butter; avocado and sunflower seeds in a salad; and a portion of mackerel with their evening meal. This leaves no room for saturated fats but the reality is that most people will also consume some in the form of butter, cheese, yogurt or milk.

In certain situations this recommendation of 1g/kg BW may need to be increased. Usually this will be linked to a training demand/ adaptation or increased energy requirements. For example, athletes who train at high altitudes and cold temperatures, such as cross-country skiers, have huge energy demands while also contending with harsh conditions. For these athletes, increasing the overall percentage of energy from fat calories may be necessary.

MICRONUTRIENTS

Don't be fooled by the prefix of 'micro' as it relates more to the fact they we only need to consume them in 'micro' amounts. They are essential nutrients. Examples are:

>>> Vitamins – A, B, C, D, E and K

>>> Minerals – calcium, iron and phosphorus

>>> Electrolytes – sodium and potassium

>>> Trace elements – iodine, zinc and magnesium

Micronutrients are essential for many metabolic processes within the body, but you can't make them yourself; you need to get them from your diet. Most function as co-enzymes or co-factors within the body – that is, they aid enzymes and proteins in their function. For example, the B vitamins are very important for carbohydrate and fat metabolism, while vitamin C, along with zinc, is important for a healthy immune system, and magnesium and calcium are needed for muscle contraction. So you can see each and every one has a huge part to play.

> **Tip**
>
> *Sources of micronutrients that you may have overlooked include herbs and spices. They are extremely high in antioxidants, which is why I always encourage their use in cooking. They also add so much flavour! You can't beat a homemade curry packed with cumin, chilli, garlic and ginger or a casserole with rosemary, thyme or sage. Whatever dish you choose, by adding herbs and spices, you will be boosting your intake of antioxidants too! See the recipe section for ideas.*

So do you need to supplement your intake to make sure you meet your requirements? The bottom line is that if you eat a well-balanced diet that includes wholegrains, vegetables, meat, fish and dairy you will have no problem in getting everything you need. In fact, in certain cases it is pointless taking on more; your daily vitamin C requirement is 60mg, which you can easily get from eating a large orange. As vitamin C is a water-soluble vitamin, you cannot store it and so any excess will just be excreted via your urine! In the same way, there have been cases reported where individuals have caused zinc toxicity by over-consuming what they need.

FACT OR FICTION?

Are certain foods really 'superfoods'?

I don't like to think of individual foods as superfoods – no one food is really able to provide all the components you need for a healthy diet. This term also gives false hope – eating a punnet of blueberries can't offset that burger you chose to have at lunchtime. That said, I do believe that individuals should aim to eat a 'super diet' high in foods that when combined will provide a diet rich in nutrients and optimize good health, meaning that cheeky burger no longer needs to be a guilty secret! No food should be off limits, but moderation, being mindful of choice and portion size are all key for those wanting to follow a 'super diet'.

So do athletes have higher requirements of micronutrients? The jury is out on this one. Some studies show that there are enhanced requirements in athletes due to an increase in damage to muscles by components known as free radicals. However, there have been no absolute links to actual improved sporting performance with a diet high in antioxidants.

So back to the original question of whether athletes have higher requirements? Technically, no, as if you are a very physically active person, you will actually be taking in more food in the form of fuel. As long as this fuel is balanced and nutrient-rich and not made up from empty calories, then you will meet your increased requirements.

Remember that all forms of fruit, vegetables, herbs and spices count. I always use frozen berries, for example, and although I prefer fresh herbs, I also have a drawer full of the dried variety. Just make sure if you are using canned varieties of fruit they are canned in just water, not sugar or syrup!

IRON

Iron is needed to make haemoglobin, which is the protein that transfers oxygen around the body. If iron levels become low, either due to a lack of intake or through excessive losses, this can manifest as iron-deficiency anaemia. An inadequate intake of iron is possible if you are following a restricted diet for weight loss, or because you are a vegan or vegetarian (see pages 47–51); excessive losses can happen during menstruation in female athletes, but have also been linked to an increased breakdown in red blood cells in some athletes, particularly those where running is involved.

Why is iron deficiency such a big deal? It becomes an issue because if there is not enough iron in the body, then the body struggles to make haemoglobin and so less oxygen can be transported around the body. This will not only make you feel pretty lousy, but will also have an impact on your overall performance. Common symptoms to look out for include:

>>> Feeling tired all the time

>>> Being short of breath, even just going up the stairs

>>> Poor performance in training

>>> Dizziness

>>> Looking pale

>>> Loss of appetite

>>> Bluish tinted dark circles around the eyes

If you have any of these symptoms, it would be worth going to talk this through with your GP, who can do a simple blood test to check your iron levels. Make sure that you get an adequate intake of diet from your diet. Red meat is the best source of iron and I always encourage athletes to aim for one portion of lean red meat a day. For vegetarians and vegans the main tip to remember is to combine vitamin C with plant-based iron-rich foods as it aids the absorption of iron. Good iron-rich foods include:

>>> Fortified cereals

>>> Dark leafy vegetables, such as spinach, kale and broccoli

>>> Lentils and other pulses

>>> Egg yolks

Tip *Don't drink tea with your iron-rich foods, or within 30 minutes of eating them, as the phytates in black tea block the absorption from these sources.*

HYDRATION - LIQUID FUEL?

Staying hydrated is essential for optimal health. Add physical activity to this equation and it's even more important as you will have more fluid losses to contend with in the form of sweat.

Being dehydrated will affect your body in many ways; most fundamentally it impairs the body's ability to regulate heat. During exercise, a rise in body temperature will lead to an elevated heart rate and this in turn makes your perceived exertion at a given training intensity feel much harder and you fatigue more quickly. Additionally, mental function is reduced, leading to negative implications for decision-making, concentration and motor control, which is needed for skill-based movements such as shooting or kicking. A symptom not often associated with dehydration is stomach discomfort; if you are dehydrated, any food you have consumed before or during training will stay in your stomach longer, leading to gastric problems.

All the above factors will have a negative effect on your exercise performance, meaning you won't get the best out of your training. This will be heightened in warmer conditions and it doesn't take much; just 2 percent dehydration (ie a loss of 1.2l/40fl oz in a 60kg/132lb athlete), can become an issue. However, the good news is this can all be combated if you learn to hydrate appropriately around your training but also on rest days.

There are no actual guidelines for fluid intake because it depends on the type and level of exercise and also varies within individuals due to:

>>> Genetics – some people innately sweat more than others

>>> Body size – larger athletes tend to sweat more than smaller athletes

>>> Fitness – fitter people sweat earlier in exercise and in larger volumes

>>> Environment – sweat losses are higher in hot, humid conditions

>>> Exercise intensity – sweat losses increase as intensity increases

So how can you make sure you are getting enough fluid? The simple answer is by checking your urine colour. The ideal is that it is pale straw in colour at all times. If it seems darker, especially before a training session, then drink! Get into the habit of monitoring your thirst levels and drink throughout the day.

I get athletes to weigh themselves before and after training sessions every now and then (and this is something you can do at home, too). This helps me to identify who has higher fluid losses and needs to be encouraged to hydrate during training sessions. So if an athlete weighs 1kg/2lb lighter after a training session and he or she has consumed 500ml (17fl oz) of fluid during the training session, it means the overall fluid loss is 1.5 litres/52fl oz, which needs to be addressed as soon as possible. In this way I help athletes to build a picture and work out how much fluid they should drink. Most athletes should aim for and should be able to tolerate between 200–300ml/7–10½fl oz every 15–20 minutes, but this may be affected by an increased intensity of exercise.

So now you know how much to drink, what should you drink? To some extent the choice is a personal one but you should take some things into consideration:

>>> When are you training?

>>> How long is your training session? Will you need fuel too?

>>> How hot is it?

For most of the time when training, water should be sufficient but many people don't like drinking water. It has been documented that for some people only having the option of water to drink will mean that they are less likely to drink. So although I'm not a massive fan of artificially sweetened drinks, when it comes to making sure you stay hydrated, I prefer that athletes drink what they know they will! So if this means they want lemon squash then so be it. If, however, you don't need to take on energy at the same time, always go for a no-added-sugar variety of drink. If you are trying to take on energy during a high-intensity or long training session, or maybe immediately before, you will benefit from something that gives you energy.

There are numerous sports drinks on the market. My advice is to choose the one you are most likely to consume. If it's hot, or you are someone who has very salty sweat losses, you will also benefit from electrolytes. If your sweat is salty, it will sting your eyes, you will be able to taste it and it will leave white residue on your clothes and body. Most branded energy drinks have both sodium (Na) and potassium (K) salts added. The normal concentration is around 10–20mmol of Na and 2–5mmol of K. These salts help to draw fluid into your body, reducing your risk of becoming dehydrated. Similarly you could add a quarter teaspoon of salt to your DIY energy drink or even use an electrolyte product.

Electrolyte products come in an array of flavours and options and they are usually in the form of a tablet or powder that you add to water. They don't provide energy, so can be useful in situations when you are training in a hot environment but don't actually need any additional energy during your training session. I have also been known to use good old rehydration salts that you can buy from the pharmacist when you have gastroenteritis. This is essentially the same product. Always follow the dosage guidelines on the packaging. In the same way if it is a short training session, I recommend drinking water and following up with foods that are higher in salt during recovery, such as soup or casserole, or salted peanuts.

SUPPLEMENTS

When you are considering the use of a supplement, it is important to consider the balance between its potential benefits – is there evidence that this product will actually boost your performance? – and also the potential risks – is this product safe to use and is it stopping me from making better food choices?

Supplements are generally classified into categories, A, B, C and D. This system ranks sports foods and supplement ingredients according to scientific evidence and other practical considerations that determine whether a product is safe, legal and effective in improving sports performance.

For the most part, the supplements of any interest to you fall into category A – sports foods, medical supplements and performance

DRUGS TESTING

When working with elite athletes, I have to be very careful about the advice I give with regards to supplements, whether that is something clinical, such as suggesting omega-3 fatty acid supplements, or more specific to training, like a protein shake or an ergogenic aid, such as bicarbonate or caffeine that has been shown to enhance performance. The reason is that at a higher level of sport, drugs testing is very common. A positive test can even come from a contaminated source of multivitamins. So when I'm advising athletes, I make sure that any product they are considering using comes from a reputable source that provides a certificate to prove that the product has been batch tested for any contaminants.

supplements (see below and opposite). These include products that have evidence to support their use in certain sporting situations and can be used by athletes as long as they are sticking to the best practice protocols. That is, athletes stick to the recommended dose. Products that fall into category B are those that have some evidence of benefits but need further studies to clarify proof of their usage – for example, fish oils, cherry juice or specific antioxidants. Products in category C have absolutely no evidence of any benefits and those in category D are generally on the banned list and should be avoided at all costs.

SPORTS FOODS

These specialized products provide a practical source of nutrients when it is impractical to consume everyday foods. They include:

>>> Sports/energy drinks

>>> Sports gels

>>> Sports confectionery, such as chews, bars and beans

>>> Liquid meal supplements

>>> Whey protein

>>> Electrolytes

MEDICAL SUPPLEMENTS

These can be used to treat clinical issues, including diagnosed nutrient deficiencies. They require individual dispensing and supervision by appropriate sports medicine/science practitioner:

>>> Iron supplements

>>> Vitamin D

>>> Other vitamin and mineral supplements – athletes must not just assume that because they are from the pharmacist, they are safe

PERFORMANCE SUPPLEMENTS

These are used to directly contribute to optimal performance. They should only be used if advice on how to use and dosage is given by a qualified sports nutritionist/practitioner. While there may be a general evidence base for these products, additional research may often be required to fine-tune protocols for individualized and event-specific use:

>>> Beetroot/beet juice

>>> Caffeine

>>> Beta-alanine

>>> Bicarbonate

>>> Creatine

So do we actually need supplements? The main difference between branded and real-food options is the ingredients list and the way in which they are marketed. Sports products can be more convenient at times but, as you can see from pages 41–44, they are not really necessary. You can generally make a real food choice, which will provide you with the same benefits, but often without the unnatural additives.

FACT
CAFFEINE

Some people can't even think about stringing a sentence together before they have had their first shot of caffeine, while others will be reduced to a nervous wreck simply from inhaling coffee fumes. So what is the deal with caffeine? For years we were told to be wary of how many caffeinated drinks we consumed daily as they had diuretic properties, resulting in dehydration. As science evolves, messages change and the truth is that a moderate consumption – 1–3 strong cups of coffee a day, 3–6 cups of tea or a can of Coke – will have no negative effect on your health.

When it comes to sports nutrition, caffeine has its own part to play. It has been used by many elite athletes as a performance-enhancing substance, but as with everything, what works for one person doesn't necessarily work for another. Individuals are either caffeine responders or non-responders. If you are someone who can drink a cup of coffee late at night and still sleep like a baby, you are a non-responder. In other words, caffeine has no effect on you at all. If, however, the opposite is true and you will be up all night, tossing and turning, you are responder. Caffeine works best as a performance enhancer in those who are responders and the suggested dose is 1–3mg/kg BW about an hour before training/competing. If you find that you respond strongly, I would suggest sticking to the lower limit of this value and definitely practise drinking this amount in training. For non-responders there is some evidence to suggest that cutting caffeine out completely for 10 days and then re-introducing it before a competition can have more enhanced effects. That said, you have to weigh up if the withdrawal symptoms are worth it or not!

My advice to athletes is that if you habitually drink caffeine then it is best not to change anything immediately before a competition.

SPORTS PRODUCT

Sports drinks eg Lucozade Sport, Gatorade, Powerade

Example ingredients list: water, glucose syrup, citric acid, acidity regulator (sodium citrate), stabilizer (acacia gum), preservative (potassium sorbate), antioxidant (ascorbic acid), sweeteners (aspartame, acesulfame K), flavouring, vitamins (niacin, panthothenic acid, B6, B12), colour (beta-carotene). Contains a source of phenylalanine.

REAL FOOD ALTERNATIVE

300ml/10½ fl oz fruit juice diluted with 200ml/7fl oz water +
¼ tsp salt

Ingredients list: pure orange juice, water, salt.

WINNING CHOICE TARGETS

>>> **Both provide 30g of carbohydrate in 500ml/17fl oz but the homemade drink has more of a natural source of sugar compared with the branded product, which is a mixture of glucose syrup and sweeteners.**

>>> **Both provide salt to aid hydration.**

>>> **The branded product will be more expensive but is usually available at competitions due to sponsorship so it's worth knowing your tolerance for these situations.**

>>> **The homemade version is cheaper but it means you have to take your own to competition situations.**

SPORTS PRODUCT
Energy gels eg TORQ, SIS, GU

Example ingredients list: maltodextrin, water, fructose, electrolytes, matric acid, natural flavour, preservative (potassium sorbate).

REAL FOOD ALTERNATIVE
6 jelly babies

Ingredients list: sugar, glucose syrup, water belatine (bovine), concentrated fruit juices* (1%), acids (citric, acetic), natural (lemon, lime, raspberry) flavourings with other natural flavourings, natural orange flavouring, natural flavourings, concentrated vegetable extracts (black carrot, spinach, stinging nettle, turmeric), colours (vegetable carbon, paprika extract, lutein) *Equivalent to 5.5% fruit.

WINNING CHOICE TARGETS

>>> **Both provide instant energy in the form of 30g carbohydrate.**

>>> **The gel may be easier to consume on higher-intensity exercise than trying to chew jelly babies.**

>>> **Jelly babies are cheaper, potentially more palatable and easier to digest, as they can be drip fed rather than taking in a concentrated amount of sugar in one hit as with a gel.**

SPORTS PRODUCT
Protein shakes eg The Simple Whey, For Goodness Shake, REGO

Example ingredients list: skimmed milk (94%), sugar flavouring, colour: beetroot, vitamin and mineral mixture (maltodextrin, magnesium hydroxide, vitamin C, zinc lactate, ferric pyrophosphate, vitamin E, vitamin B3, sodium selenite, biotin, manganese sulphate, vitamin B5, vitamin A, copper sulphate, vitamins B6, B9, D3, B1, B2, potassium iodide), stabilisers: carrageenan, guar gum.

REAL FOOD ALTERNATIVE

Flavoured milk, homemade milkshakes such as Recovery Hot Chocolate (see page 277) or Mocha Shake (see page 277) and smoothies such as Tropical Smoothie (see page 276) or Summer Fruit Smoothie (see page 182)

Example ingredients list (for shop-bought flavoured milk): semi-skimmed milk, skimmed milk, sugar (4.5%), strawberry juice from concentrate (1%), natural flavouring, stabiliser: gellan Gum, colour: beta-carotene

WINNING CHOICE TARGETS

>>> **The majority of protein shakes are based on milk – see opposite.**

>>> **Whey protein is an isolated milk protein so when taken alone will be in a higher concentration. The theory is that because it is absorbed into the body more quickly, it is more readily digestible and allows for better muscle protein synthesis (the repair and rebuilding of muscle).**

>>> **Some studies demonstrate benefits of whey over milk but these gains are not significant enough to warrant the use of whey over milk.**

>>> **Protein shakes are extremely expensive: 500ml/17fl oz For Goodness Shake is five times more expensive than 500ml/17fl oz chocolate milk.**

>>> **Some protein shakes have more protein than recommended or needed whereas 500ml/17fl oz flavoured milk provides 20g of protein.**

>>> **Many protein shakes are devoid of carbohydrate, which may be useful in some training situations but not many.**

>>> **Protein shakes have a higher risk attached with regards to testing. They are easy to contaminate with prohibited substances, especially if they have added products such as growth hormone or creatine.**

>>> **Protein shakes may be more convenient in certain situations.**

SPORTS PRODUCT

Sports bars eg Clif Bar, PowerBar, Promax

Example ingredients list: organic brown rice syrup, organic rolled oats, soy rice crisps (soy protein isolate, rice flour, rice starch, barley malt extract), organic roasted soybeans, organic soy flour), dried apricots (apricots, evaporated cane juice, rice flour, citric acid, ascorbic acid, organic oat fibre, inulin (chicory extract), organic milled flaxseed, organic oat bran, organic psyllium), organic cane syrup, dried apricots, organic date paste, organic sunflower oil, natural flavours, lemon juice concentrate, citric acid, sea salt, coloured with annatto.

REAL FOOD ALTERNATIVE

Real food options such as Chia Charge and Nookie Bars or recipes from this book such as Nut Butter Squares (see page 266), Dark Chocolate and Ginger Muffins (see page 260) or Sweet Potato Brownies (see page 264); jam/yeast extract sandwiches or dried fruit and nuts.

Example ingredients list (for a real-food sports bar): oats, butter, demerara sugar, golden syrup, chia seeds (9%), sea salt flakes.

WINNING CHOICE TARGETS

>>> **In a situation where it is possible to eat, such as on a long bike ride/hike/trail run, real food options are always better.**

SPECIAL DIETARY CONSIDERATIONS

Every year there is an influx of 'wonder diets' – high-fat, low-carbohydrate, gluten-free – the promise of 'the next big' thing that will bring potential health benefits, the body beautiful or athletic prowess, but are they the real deal or just another form of faddism? Not surprisingly, people become confused by this array of different diets and I'm often asked what are the best foods to eat for optimal performance gains. Some of these diets are backed by scientific studies, while others seem to appear from thin air. That is why it is important to use regulated practitioners, such as dietitians or registered nutritionists, who have to ensure that all their advice is accurate and evidence based.

A GLUTEN-FREE DIET

In recent years there has been a real trend toward individuals wanting to follow a gluten-free diet. Gluten has become a huge subject of controversy, with many blaming it for symptoms such as bloating, fatigue and even joint pain. Many high-profile individuals, including athletes such as tennis player Ivan Djokovic, report benefits, particularly in performance, since removing gluten from their diets.

Gluten is the protein found within wheat and related grains, including barley and rye. It is therefore found in foods such as bread, pasta and cereals, but also in sausages and beer. For most individuals, gluten does not pose a problem. The body has the ability to break it down, as with other proteins, absorb it and utilize it as necessary. Evidence of the benefits of a gluten-free diet for those individuals where it is not medically necessary is very thin on the ground.

Ultimately, if individuals want to follow a gluten-free diet, it is their choice. They may indeed feel more energized and less bloated, but this could be due to them being more mindful of nutritional choices. We should all eat less white bread, biscuits/cookies, cakes, white pasta etc and by following a gluten-free diet these foods will automatically be removed. However, do not be fooled into thinking that a gluten-free diet is healthier. There is a lack of wholegrain gluten-free products and they also tend to be higher in fat and sugar in order to make them more palatable. That said, there are people who need to remove gluten from their diet for medical reasons.

COELIAC DISEASE

Coeliac disease is an autoimmune condition, meaning the body's immune system attacks and destroys healthy body tissue in error. It affects the small intestine, causing it to become damaged and unable to absorb vital nutrients such as calcium, iron and energy from food. The symptoms are usually weight loss, extreme fatigue due to iron deficiency, bloating, and very frequent bowel movements. Due to an inability to absorb calcium, those who have coeliac disease may also be at an increased risk of osteoporosis, which makes your bones weak putting you at a greater risk of fractures and breaks if you fall.

Coeliac disease is usually confirmed by taking blood tests and gut biopsies. The individual will then be put on a strict gluten-free diet, which they will need to comply with for life.

WHEAT ALLERGY

A small percentage of individuals suffer from wheat allergy. Unlike the symptoms for coeliac disease (see above), wheat allergy tends to affect the skin. There is usually an immediate allergic reaction that causes itchy skin, itchy eyes and there may even be swelling of both eyes and throat. A wheat allergy is usually diagnosed by skin-prick testing and the individual will need to remove all wheat from their diet.

THE PROMISE OF PERFORMANCE GAINS

Some claim that a gluten-free diet can improve athletic performance. Scientifically there is no proof of this, unless of course you have coeliac disease or have been diagnosed with a true wheat allergy. However, being more mindful of your food choices and tailoring your nutrition to your training sessions can help. Including complex carbohydrates (see page 19), with or without gluten, when you actually need them and keeping foods high in sugar to a minimum are strategies that will definitely result in improvements to your health and performance.

Fuelling your sport is not about the inclusion or removal of one particular food or food type. It is about achieving the correct overall balance and tailoring your nutritional intake to your needs. Finding the correct balance of macronutrients – carbohydrates, protein and fats; micronutrients – vitamins and minerals, including antioxidants, as well as staying fully hydrated all play a part. Understanding the role of these individual components and how to apply this information is key to ensuring a healthy balanced diet, and ensuring the elements work together to become effective training foods.

THE VEGETARIAN AND VEGAN ATHLETE

Many athletes consider the move to a more plant-based diet. Vegetarians eat no animal flesh, but will consume eggs or dairy. Vegans don't consume any foods of animal origin.

The reasons for choosing either a vegetarian or vegan diet could be one of many:

>>> Cultural or religious beliefs

>>> Moral beliefs relating to animal welfare

>>> Health benefits

>>> Environmental issues

So can a plant-based diet really be practical and sufficient for long-term athletic success? The answer is of course, yes, but more time and consideration may be needed to plan meals and recovery to ensure that you are meeting all your nutritional requirements for both macro- and micro-nutrients (see page 31).

It is often thought that vegetarian and vegan diets cannot support a heavy training load, with many individuals believing that protein requirements cannot be met. A vegetarian diet can indeed provide all essential nutrients to support intense daily training and competition needs in athletes. However, there are still several dietary challenges that need to be addressed but with the right information to hand, a vegetarian/vegan diet can be an excellent choice.

By becoming familiar with vegetarian protein alternatives, you can create some nutritious and creative meals/snacks, such as the Banana and Nut Butter Sandwich (see page 267) or Harissa and Cumin Hummus (see page 271) with raw veg sticks.

GOOD PROTEIN SOURCES

For vegetarians only:

>>> Eggs

>>> Low-fat dairy products, including milk, cheese and yogurt, particularly Greek yogurt

>>> Whey protein

For both vegans and vegetarians:

>>> Pulses e.g. chickpeas, kidney beans, mung beans, black-eyed peas, lentils

>>> Tofu

>>> Soya – all products

>>> Quorn

>>> Nuts and nut butters

>>> Seeds

In some cases, where training volumes are very high, it might be difficult to meet energy requirements due to the fact that a vegetarian/vegan diet can be high in fibre and bulk, filling you up more quickly and leaving less space for energy-dense foods. Indeed it has been observed that vegans in particular, and those vegetarians who don't just replace meat with cheese or high-fat meat alternatives often weigh less. This can be advantageous in some sports but it is always important to ensure that you have sufficient energy to meet your training needs. By using the guidelines in this book, and adapting them with suitable vegetarian/vegan options, you can be sure to meet all your training food needs.

This should not be too problematic for the vegetarians amongst you, as many of the recovery options include low-fat milk or Greek yogurt. It can, however, be a little trickier for vegans. Although there has been a rise in suitable dairy alternatives becoming available, many options such as almond, coconut, oat, rice or hazelnut milk, are actually very low in both carbohydrate and protein. The table below compares the nutritional content of almond, soya and skimmed cow's milk.

	Unsweetened almond milk	Unsweetened soya milk	Skimmed cow's milk
Energy/Kcals	26	44	66
Carbohydrate/g	0.2	0.2	10
Protein/g	0.8	4	7
Fat/g	2.2	2.4	0.2

TABLE 1.3 Nutritional content of milks (per 200ml/7fl oz)

As we know, the combination of carbohydrate and protein in a liquid form is one of the best ways to recover from a hard, high-intensity training session, while having protein in an easily digestible form is also important around a strength training session.

From Table 1.3, it is very clear that both almond and soya milk are lacking vital carbohydrates but this can be addressed by adding banana and honey to provide carbohydrate from a recovery perspective. However, the low levels of protein, particularly in almond milk, doesn't make this a suitable recovery option. Again a vegan could get around this by introducing additional protein. I know some vegan athletes who use hemp or pea protein powders. I often recommend adding ground almonds as 25g serving provides 6.5g of protein but ideally I would suggest that vegan athletes aim to use soya milk in preference to other dairy alternatives.

In the same way, making sure that you take on 0.25g/kg BW protein 4–6 times a day from whole food protein sources (see list opposite) will ensure that your training needs are met. Additionally, proteins such as sesame seeds, sunflower seeds, tofu and pumpkin seeds, are rich sources of BCAA (branched chain amino acids – see page 101), which can be useful to include in the hour before strength training sessions.

There are a few other nutrients that may be more difficult to obtain from a vegetarian or vegan diet:

>>> **Iron and zinc:** Although very abundant in plant sources, these nutrients are not always readily available. Beans, wholegrains, nuts, and seeds

have a high zinc content but these foods are also high in phytate, which inhibits absorption of both iron and zinc. The bioavailability of zinc is enhanced by dietary protein but could potentially be inhibited by supplements that also contain folic acid, iron, calcium, copper and magnesium. Zinc supplementation or a multivitamin/multi-mineral containing zinc is a wise choice for vegan athletes, but be aware of the interactions stated above. For those athletes who would prefer to consume zinc more naturally, pumpkin seeds and hemp seeds are very good sources.

>>> **Calcium**: This should not be an issue for vegetarian or vegan athletes as long as you continue to consume 3–4 servings of dairy or soya products daily. Additional non-dairy sources of calcium include:

>> Nuts, particularly almonds and cashews

>> Tofu

>> Sesame seeds and tahini

>> Chickpeas

>> Dark green leafy vegetables (will be needed in large volumes)

>>> **Vitamin B12**: This is only available in animal sources, so most vegetarians who consume eggs or dairy produce will still meet their requirements. However, this is a nutrient that will be completely void in a vegan diet and needs to be supplemented. It is an essential nutrient required for correct functioning of the nervous system and formation of red blood cells.

>>> **Omega-3 Fatty Acids**: The omega-3 fatty acids EPA, eicosapentaenoic acid, and DHA, docosahexaenoic acid, are important for brain and heart function and in athletes they seem to have a role in reducing inflammation and oxidative stress. The best source of EPA and DHA is oily fish such as salmon and mackerel, which won't form part of a vegetarian and vegan diet. However, another omega-3 fatty acid, ALA, alpha-linolenic acid, can be used by the body to make EPA and DHA. Good sources of ALA include:

>> Linseeds/flaxseeds

>> Chia seeds

>> Walnuts and walnut oil

>> Hemp seeds

That said, the amount of ALA obtained from these sources may not be sufficient to meet the levels in order to produce EPA and DHA. It may be useful for vegetarian and vegan athletes to include an algae-based omega-3 fatty acid supplement, as well as include good intakes of the above sources of dietary ALA, to ensure that sufficient levels are met for the conversion.

RECOVERY NUTRITION

So, as important it is to get training nutrition right, it is equally, if not slightly more important to get recovery nutrition spot on. To consistently produce a high level of performance, day after day, week after week, month after month, your recovery nutrition has to be optimal.

If training is the stimulus, which you have correctly fuelled, recovery food is now needed in response to this stimulus to make sure that the body can convert this stimulus to gains.

Timing of recovery is very important and it differs according to how you train. The majority of my athletes tend to compete at a fairly high level, even within university sport. This means that they tend to have more than one training session a day. For some of you training for an event such as a triathlon where there are three disciplines to cover, it may be logistically the only way you can fit all your training in.

The same principle about recovery nutrition will also apply if you have training sessions in less than 12 hours of each other. For example, a late-night training session, followed by an early-morning training session, regardless of what sport you are doing. The recovery period is short between sessions, so to help your body resynthesize glycogen stores in preparation for the next session, your recovery food should be taken within 15–30 minutes of finishing your training. Ideally it should also be in a liquid form, with a mixture of fast-release carbohydrate and easily digestible protein. This is why milk and milk products have become popular as recovery choices. The combination of carbohydrate and protein in an easy digestible form means your muscles receive the building blocks they need to help repair and recover them quickly and efficiently before your next training session.

So what if you don't have another training session for 24 hours? Recovery nutrition is still important, and there is still an important window to fill, but you only need to have the recovery food within two hours of finishing your training, which may well fall at your next meal.

What and how much you should eat will depend on the intensity of your training session. If you have had a high-intensity session, the recommended guidelines in sports nutrition are 1–1.2g/kg BW of carbohydrate with 0.25g/kg BW protein. So for a 60kg/132lb athlete who has just finished a high-intensity 60-minute turbo session, this will mean between 60–72g of carbohydrate and 15g of protein. This will help to replenish glycogen stores, enhance recovery and help that all-important adaptation (see page 98). I want to point out here that the addition of the protein helps to compensate if you don't quite meet the upper end of the carbohydrate intake. So what would this look like as food choices? For a recovery between two sessions, I would opt for something like:

>>> Mocha Shake (see page 277), which provides 10g per serving

If it was a meal option then:

>>> Scrambled Egg Pitta (see page 192), which provides19g per serving

You would then repeat this recommendation throughout the day at 2–3 hourly intervals.

If it has been a lower-intensity session and you are not training again for 24 hours, stick with the 0.25g/kg BW protein but you will need to adjust your carbohydrate throughout the day. On page 18, we looked at the amount of carbohydrate you need daily according to the activity type, level and duration. It is important to ensure that you meet this requirement but there are no specifics on when.

So if you have done a light activity your overall carbohydrate requirement for the day will be 3g/kg BW if you are a female and 5g/kg BW if you are a male. As an example, for a 60kg/132lb female athlete, this translates to 180g of carbohydrate for a day.

As it is a light activity, you may have chosen to do this in a fasted state first thing in the morning. After your session you will want breakfast. As long as your breakfast has 15g of protein, it does not matter whether you choose to have carbohydrate with it or not. However, you must make sure that you meet your carbohydrate requirement through the day. I normally suggest that individuals distribute their carbohydrate allowance among their other meals, using nutrient-dense varieties such as root vegetables, legumes and pulses to prevent blood sugars from fluctuating and you from succumbing to the biscuit barrel/cookie jar mid-afternoon! Don't forget, on these lighter carbohydrate days, making good choices means that your allowance will go further.

YOUR METABOLISM

How the body converts food to fuel relies upon several different energy pathways. Having a basic understanding of these systems will help you train and eat efficiently to ensure improved sports performance. We have already discussed how sports nutrition involves an understanding of how nutrients such as carbohydrate, fat, and protein contribute to the fuel supply needed by the body to perform exercise. These nutrients get converted to energy in the form of adenosine triphosphate (ATP) via different metabolic pathways; ATP is a molecule within cells used for energy transfer and it is this energy released by the breakdown of ATP that allows muscle cells to contract. As already mentioned, carbohydrates, proteins and fats have unique properties and so follow different metabolic pathways in order to be converted to ATP.

ENERGY PATHWAYS

The body cannot easily store ATP and what is stored gets used up within a few seconds, so it is necessary to continually create ATP during exercise. There are two major ways the body converts nutrients to energy:

>>> Aerobic metabolism (with oxygen)

>>> Anaerobic metabolism (without oxygen)

Most often it's a combination of energy systems that supply the fuel needed for exercise, with the intensity and duration of the exercise determining which method gets used when.

AEROBIC METABOLISM

Aerobic metabolism fuels most of the energy needed for long duration activity, that is any activity that is over 2 minutes. It uses oxygen to convert nutrients (carbohydrates, fats, and protein) to ATP. This system is a bit slower than the anaerobic systems because it relies on the circulatory system to transport oxygen to the working muscles before it creates ATP. Aerobic metabolism is used primarily during endurance exercise, which is generally less intense and can continue for long periods of time.

ANAEROBIC METABOLISM

Anaerobic metabolism is your body's way of producing energy quickly, without the need for oxygen. There are 2 different pathways for this:

1 > The ATP-CP energy pathway, also known as the phosphate system, supplies about 10 seconds worth of energy and is used for short bursts of exercise such as a 100m sprint. This pathway doesn't require any oxygen to create ATP. It first uses up any ATP stored in the muscle (about 2–3 seconds worth) and then it uses creatine phosphate (CP) to resynthesize ATP until the CP runs out (another 6–8 seconds). Creatine phosphate is a molecule found in the muscles, which serves as a rapidly available and transportable reserve of energy. Once all available ATP and CP are used, the body will move on to either aerobic or glycolysis to continue to create ATP in order to fuel the exercise.

2 > Glycolysis is the predominant energy system used for all-out exercise lasting from 30 seconds to about 2 minutes, such as in events like 400/800m, and is the second-fastest way to resynthesize ATP.

During glycolysis, carbohydrate, either as glucose within the blood or glucose that has been converted from glycogen stores, is broken down through a series of chemical reactions to form pyruvate. For every molecule of glucose broken down to pyruvate through glycolysis, two molecules of usable ATP are produced. Two molecules of useable ATP is enough to fuel an all-out sprint of up to 40 seconds. Therefore, very little energy is produced through this pathway, but the trade-off is that you get the energy quickly.

During exercise an athlete will move through all these metabolic pathways. As exercise begins, ATP is produced via anaerobic metabolism as there is an oxygen debt/lag. With an increase in breathing and heart rate, there is more oxygen available and aerobic metabolism begins and continues until the lactate threshold is reached.

LACTATE THRESHOLD

'Lactate' or lactic acid is a unique metabolic product produced by the body in response to exercise that indicates your potential for athletic performance. At rest your lactate levels are 1mmol/l. During exercise, muscles use glucose as a fuel source – this glucose molecule is converted to another molecule known as pyruvate which, when combined with oxygen, acts as an energy source, in the form of ATP in the muscles, as we have seen.

As exercise intensity increases, the amount of oxygen available to the muscles decreases and some pyruvate is broken down into lactate and Hydrogen (H) ions, which start to increase the acidity within the muscle. At first the rest of the body is able to buffer this acidity, preventing the accumulation of lactic acid and H ions and the onset of rapid fatigue; however, as exercise intensity increases the body's ability to buffer this acid accumulation becomes compromised and an increase in the blood lactate level occurs. This is known as your lactate threshold and occurs when blood lactate levels reach 4mmol/l, causing that all too familiar 'burn' and fatigue. Although it is the rise in H ions that causes an increase in acidity, it is termed your 'lactate threshold' as it is lactate levels that are being measured in the lab during an exercise test and determine at which pace this threshold occurs.

Many athletes like to work at their 'threshold' as it offers a good determination of the maximum exercise speed that an endurance athlete can sustain for a long period of time (typically greater than 20–30 minutes, which is useful to know when trying to work out your threshold without having to go to the expense of an exercise test). Training that is specifically tailored to increase this 'lactate threshold' will therefore result in faster race times. It is also thought to be one of the best indicators of endurance performance. Generally athletes whose 'lactate threshold' occurs at a higher speed will be faster in an endurance event as they have a higher tolerance to this accumulation of H ions and delay the onset fatigue. So training at this threshold is almost always accompanied by improvements in race performance for endurance events.

FUELLING THE ENERGY SYSTEMS

Nutrients get converted to ATP based upon the intensity and duration of activity, with carbohydrate as the main nutrient fuelling exercise of a moderate to high intensity, and fat providing energy during exercise that occurs at a lower intensity. Fat is a great source of fuel for endurance events as it can produce energy for several hours or even days in the presence of oxygen, but it is simply not adequate for high-intensity exercise such as sprints intervals or even holding a 'race pace', which will be just below your lactate threshold.

So in general terms, as exercise intensity increases, carbohydrate metabolism takes over. It is more efficient than fat metabolism, but has limited energy stores. This stored carbohydrate (glycogen) can fuel about 2 hours of moderate- to high-level exercise. After that, glycogen depletion occurs (stored carbohydrates are used up) and if that fuel isn't replaced athletes may hit the wall or 'bonk'. An athlete can continue moderate- to high-intensity exercise for longer by simply replenishing carbohydrate stores during exercise. This is why it is critical to eat easily digestible carbohydrates during moderate exercise that lasts more than a few hours. If you don't take in enough carbohydrate, you will be forced to reduce your intensity and tap back into fat metabolism to fuel activity.

If exercise intensity increases further, carbohydrate metabolism efficiency drops off dramatically and anaerobic metabolism takes over. This is because your body cannot take in and distribute oxygen quickly enough to use either fat or carbohydrate metabolism easily. In fact, carbohydrate can produce nearly 20 times more energy (in the form of ATP) per gram when metabolized in the presence of adequate oxygen than when generated in the oxygen-starved, anaerobic environment that occurs during intense efforts (sprinting).

With appropriate training, these energy systems adapt and become more efficient and allow greater exercise duration at higher intensity.

MUSCLE FIBRE TYPES

Skeletal muscle is made up of bundles of individual muscle fibres called myocytes. Each myocyte contains many myofibrils, which are strands of proteins (actin and myosin) that can grab on to each other and pull. This shortens the muscle and causes muscle contraction. It is generally accepted that muscle fibre types can be broken down into two main types:

>>> Slow-twitch (Type I) muscle fibres

>>> Fast-twitch (Type II) muscle fibres. Fast-twitch fibres can be further categorized into Type IIa and Type IIb fibres

These distinctions seem to influence how muscles respond to training and physical activity, and each fibre type is unique in its ability to contract in a certain way. Human muscles contain a genetically determined mixture of both slow and fast fibre types. On average, we have about 50 percent slow-twitch and 50 per cent fast-twitch fibres in most of the muscles used for movement.

SLOW-TWITCH (TYPE I)

Slow-twitch fibres are more efficient at using oxygen to generate more fuel (ATP) for continuous, extended muscle contractions over a long time. They fire more slowly than fast-twitch fibres and can go for a long time before they fatigue and so are very useful to endurance athletes.

FAST-TWITCH (TYPE II)

Because fast-twitch fibres use anaerobic metabolism to create fuel, they are much better at generating short bursts of strength or speed than slow muscles. However, they fatigue more quickly. Fast-twitch fibres generally produce the same amount of force per contraction as slow muscles, but they get their name because they are able to fire more rapidly. Having a higher percentage of fast-twitch fibres can be an asset to sprint/power athletes, as they need to generate a lot of force quickly.

FIBRE TYPE AND PERFORMANCE

Our muscle fibre type may influence what sports we are naturally good at or whether we are fast or strong. This is usually the case in elite athletes who tend to fall into sports that match their genetic makeup; sprinters have been shown to possess about 80 percent fast-twitch fibres, while marathon runners tend to have 80 percent slow-twitch fibres.

So this poses the question, can you change the distribution of your fibre type to suit your sport? Can a 50m freestyle swimmer be just as good as an open-water endurance swimmer? This is a huge area of research but there are still no conclusive answers. There is some evidence demonstrating that human skeletal muscle may switch fibre types from 'fast' to 'slow' due to training but further studies are needed to confirm this.

BODY COMPOSITION

In sports nutrition, it is more helpful to look at body composition than body mass/weight alone. The human body is composed of a variety of different components:

>>> Lean tissues, such as muscle, bone, and organs, are metabolically active

>>> Fat or adipose tissue are not metabolically active

Together these components of fat mass and fat-free mass (lean tissue) make up an individual's total body weight. However, in sports nutrition it is more useful to look at the proportion of these individual components and this is known as body composition. Standing on most scales can tell you what you weigh but it can't help you to determine how much of this weight is muscle or fat. This is also why BMI (Body Mass Index) has recently been under scrutiny. For example, a 103kg/230lb rugby player who is 1.83m/6ft tall would have a BMI of 30. This would actually put him in the obese category of most standard weight charts. However, if we were to look at his body composition and find that he had a body fat percentage of 12, this would be completely acceptable for a male athlete.

HOW DO YOU MEASURE BODY COMPOSITION?

There are many methods but the technique that I tend to employ is using skinfold calipers. This instrument pinches the fold of skin to pull it away from the underlying muscle so only the skin and fat tissue is being held. Measurements are usually taken at seven sites. The skinfold thickness is measured in millimetres. The total measurements from all seven sites will provide a value that can then be used to convert to a percentage of body fat.

If a trained practitioner completes this process, it has been shown to be 98 percent accurate and is the gold standard choice of most sports nutritionists and physiologists due to its relatively low cost.

Bioelectrical impedance testing is now becoming very popular in some gyms and clinics as it is easy, quick and doesn't involve sending practitioners away to be trained in taking skinfold measurements. However, the accuracy of these machines/scales needs to be questioned as values are affected by hydration levels, food intake and skin temperature.

A female client came to see me about three months ago. She had been told that her body fat percentage was 37 after bioelectrical impedance testing. When I measured her body composition using skinfold calipers, her actual result was 29 percent.

WHAT IS THE IDEAL BODY COMPOSITION?

This will vary depending on gender and age but the average acceptable range for males is 15–18 percent body fat and for females it is 22–25 percent for general health.

In the athlete population, the figure tends to be significantly lower. In males it will be 6–15 percent and in females, 12–20 percent. Dropping below 6 percent in males and 12 percent in female athletes is not acceptable and can be detrimental to health and performance. Indeed studies have shown there is no advantage in performance when male athletes drop below 8 percent or females below 14 percent. Body composition will vary from sport to sport; for example in cycling typical values are 5–15 percent for males and 15–20 percent for females. In swimming males range between 9–12 percent and females 14–24 percent; for marathon runners males fall between 5–11 percent and females 10–15 percent.

So while low levels of body fat seem to be related to improved performance, body composition alone is not a great predictor of sports success. For example a rugby player needs to have enough body mass (lean and fat weight) to generate high forces and avoid injury.

The key to being successful in your chosen sport is to train well, fuel your training correctly and, in most cases, this generally leads to favourable body composition to enhance performance.

Summary

>>> Fuelling with the right foods can make a huge difference to sports performance

>>> Carbohydrate is the body's primary fuel. Stored as glycogen in our muscles, it can be converted quickly into energy

>>> Fat can also be an important fuel source for endurance activities – bodies can become 'fat adapted' to take energy from fat stores, but this is a slower process

>>> Protein is made up of amino acids – the building blocks of the body – and is essential to recovery

>>> Micronutrients, as well as iron, are also essential for the body's functions

>>> Sports nutrition can be tailored to special diets, such as gluten-free, vegetarian or vegan diets

>>> Nutrition is as important for recovery as it is for performance, replacing lost resources and preparing the body for the next training session

>>> There are different energy pathways for metabolizing fuel depending on the intensity and duration of your exercise

CHAPTER 2:
TRAINING THE ROAD TO VICTORY

TRAINING TO PERFORM

You are likely to have chosen your sport because you have a natural aptitude for it or are particularly enthusiastic about it, but neither inherent ability or an avid interest will necessarily make you excel. In order to be really good at your sport, you not only have to train but train in the *right* way.

The term 'training' can mean so many things. For some of you it will be about increasing your stamina over an increasing distance; for others it will be about increasing your speed. You might train using a combination of speed, core, strength and endurance sessions or you might use only one or perhaps two of those techniques. Some of you will go with active rest days (see page 95), while others might take whole days off altogether. Whether your sport is running, cycling, swimming or team-based, you probably know that training is fundamental to your performance, but what do all the different kinds of training actually mean and how do they relate to you and your sport? Where does nutrition fit in? In this chapter we are going to:

>>> Explore the different types of training and how they will help your body to become more efficient for your particular event

>>> Ensure you get the best out of your training by looking at your body's fuel demands for each type of training, and for rest days, too

This chapter also includes meal plans, using the recipes at the back of the book, to help you make the right choices around your chosen sport, as well as the level of intensity you will be exercising at that day. There are 10 different meal plan days for each intensity level of exercise. So for example, if you are having a high-intensity day of training, where you will have higher requirements for carbohydrate than on a low-intensity day, select a meal plan from this section that fits in with your day. The plans also take into consideration the timing of your training, helping to fuel your muscles beforehand and recover appropriately after your workout.

TYPES OF SPORT

In Chapter 1 we learned how the body uses fuel to create energy through aerobic and anaerobic metabolism (see pages 53–5). Take another look at those pages now if you need to because the information in them is fundamental to understanding how to train for maximum competitive efficiency.

Sports fall into three broad categories:

>>> Endurance – running any distance over 1,500m; cycling; triathlon

>>> Sprint/power – running from 100–1,500m; 50m freestyle swimming; tennis

>>> Team sports – requiring a mixture of both speed/power and
    endurance, such as football, netball and rugby

To train for and excel in each of these types of sports, you need to understand what fuelling mechanisms the body uses for each. In endurance sports, training will involve building your aerobic fitness but also working to maintain a given intensity over long distances. For sprint sports, the majority of the training will focus on increasing anaerobic fitness, speed and power. The training for team sports will involve increasing your aerobic fitness for endurance, as well as working on your anaerobic fitness for power/speed, and not forgetting the skills/drills to help with match play.

When training for any sport, keep your goal in mind, as this will determine what key training sessions you need to include and how to fuel them appropriately. So, for example, if your goal is to run a personal best time in a marathon, the key energy system involved is going to be the aerobic system. You will definitely include faster paced training sessions, but you will not benefit from including 100m sprint repetitions, which will actually enhance your anaerobic ATP-CP energy system. Think back to Chapter 1 where we looked at energy systems, and remember that the ATP-CP system only provides energy for events that last under 20 seconds. A marathon is going to take significantly longer and so a large majority of training needs to be focused on improving your aerobic system.

Another example is football. From the table below you can see that 50 percent of the energy provided comes from the Anaerobic ATP-CP system, 20 percent from Anaerobic glycolysis and 30 percent from the Aerobic system. Football involves multiple sprints within an endurance framework, therefore training will involve improving all three of these energy systems. The table below demonstrates further examples to summarize this:

Activity	% contribution of ATP-PC energy system	% contribution of glycolysis	% contribution of oxidative/aerobic energy system
Track events such as 100m and 200m sprints	90	10	0
400m sprint	17	48	35
1,500m	4	20	76
Marathon	0	1	99
Football	50	20	30
Tennis	70	20	10
Swimming 50m freestyle	40	55	5
Swimming (distance)	10	20	70
Skiing	33	33	33

TABLE 2.1 Contribution from each energy system for different sports

TRAINING INTENSITY

There are also three levels of intensity when training::

>>> Low

>>> Moderate

>>> High

In a given week, most sports will require you to cover a combination of training at different intensities, depending on your overall goal.

So, for example, the training plan for someone training for an endurance event, such as long-distance running or swimming, may be as follows:

>>> Monday – low-intensity training for 60–90 mins

>>> Tuesday – high-intensity intervals (60 mins) at lactate threshold (see pages 55–6) or just above

>>> Wednesday – rest day

>>> Thursday – high-intensity continuous training (45–60 mins) at lactate threshold or just below to emulate race pace

>>> Friday – low-intensity training for 60–90 mins

>>> Saturday – moderate-intensity training for 60 mins

>>> Sunday – low-intensity training for longer than 90 mins

An example of a training schedule for a netball player might be:

>>> Monday – gym-based weights

>>> Tuesday – high-intensity reps (60 mins) above lactate threshold (see pages 55–6) to train anaerobic system

>>> Wednesday – moderate/high-intensity match play (60 mins)

>>> Thursday – rest day

>>> Friday – high-intensity reps (60 mins) above lactate threshold to train anaerobic system

>>> Saturday – gym-based weights

>>> Sunday – moderate- to high-intensity match play (up to 2 hours)

Knowing and being able to gauge the intensity of your exercise is important to help you determine the amounts and types of fuel you require for a given training session. The most commonly used scale is based on the research of Gunnar Borg, a researcher and lecturer at Stockholm University in the 1970s. It is sometimes called the Borg Scale. This measures your rate of perceived effort in a scale (RPE) from 1–10 where 1 is no effort and 10 is maximal effort.

Rating	Description
0	Nothing at all
0.5	Very, very light
1	Very light
2	Fairly light
3	Moderate
4	Somewhat hard
5	Hard
6	
7	Very hard
8	
9	
10	Very, very hard (maximal)

TABLE 2.2 The Borg Scale

The higher the intensity – anything above 7 out of 10 – the more important it is that carbohydrate is available as the main fuel source to maintain that intensity for a given period. If you are going to do something like a spinning class, a sparring session or run intervals, it is essential that you have consumed sufficient carbohydrate beforehand so you can hold the high-intensity nature of these training sessions.

Remember, carbohydrate is rapidly and easily converted to glucose to supply the working muscle with sufficient energy to maintain this high-intensity exercise. If you do not consume sufficient carbohydrate, your body will look to break down fat stores into glucose. However, this process occurs at a much slower rate, which means that glucose is not delivered fast enough to the working muscle and so exercise intensity needs to be reduced. It also explains why there is less need for carbohydrate as fuel when exercising at a lower intensity.

We will look at the benefits and nutritional implications of training at each of these intensities later in this chapter. The table below is a quick-reference guide:

High intensity (more than 7/10 RPE or 70% or higher of your maximum heart rate) Main fuel used = carbohydrate	Moderate intensity (6/10 RPE or 60–70% of your maximum heart rate) Fuel used = carbohydrate + fat	Low intensity (5/10 or 50% or lower of your maximum heart rate) Fuel used if done in fasted state = fat
Spinning/turbo (20–60 mins)	Long bike ride (longer than 90 mins)	Yoga/Pilates/body balance
Running intervals (20–60 mins)	Steady/long run (longer than 90 mins)	Recovery run (up to 60 mins)
Some positions in team sport matches such as football, hockey, netball (60 mins)	Some positions in team sport, drills/skill session such as football, hockey, netball (60 mins)	Gardening/ housework such as hoovering, dusting, mopping floors (60 mins)
Swimming intervals/efforts (20–60 mins)	Continuous swimming but not all-out effort (45–60 mins)	Walking slowly/leisurely (up to 60 mins)
Circuits with very little rest periods between stations (60 mins)	Walking fast or up a hill but still able to have a conversation (60 mins)	
Boxing /sparring/skipping (20–60 mins)		

TABLE 2.3 Training intensities for specific sports and activities

This table is just a guide. Only you can really determine how hard you are training or are proposing to train; for example, some argue that there are types of yoga that are not low intensity because they can really get your heart pumping. In a similar way, an activity that is low intensity for one person may actually feel like a moderate to hard intensity to another – it will depend on the individual's starting point. So someone new to exercise may find walking at a brisk pace a high-intensity exercise, whereas a seasoned marathon runner will find this low intensity. As previously stated, in most sports there will be training sessions held at all intensities.

LOW-INTENSITY TRAINING

This will feel like 5/10 or around 50 percent of your maximum heart rate if you train using a heart-rate monitor. Whether you are cycling, swimming or running, this is an easy pace; you should feel fairly comfortable and be able to have a conversation easily and, to some extent, feel almost like you have more energy when you finish!

LOW-INTENSITY TRAINING FOR RECOVERY

We know that working at a high intensity increases the acidity within the muscle and for some people it can take over 24 hours for levels to return back to normal. In some training plans, low-intensity training is often used as a recovery session, 12–24 hours after a high-intensity session to help return this acidity back to normal. By working at a low intensity, the body can increase its uptake of oxygen, which in turn can help buffer this acid. So, for example, if you have completed a high-intensity turbo session, your body will still be fatigued up to 24 hours later. By doing a low-intensity bike ride for 20–60 minutes as your next training session, you will give your body a chance to recover, while still working your aerobic system but at a level where there is no additional stress on your body. This format of alternative day training sessions also helps to reduce the risk of injury and illness as your body is not continually pushed to a maximal level.

Tip
Cyclists taking part in the Tour de France often train on a stationary bike after they have finished their stage. It is an attempt to reduce acidity, helping the muscles recover as best they can before the next day of maximal riding at a high intensity.

FUELLING LOW-INTENSITY TRAINING

At this intensity, it is essential to stay hydrated. A lot of people are unaware that the 'heavy leg' feeling you sometimes get is caused by dehydration. Try to ensure that you are hydrated before you start exercising. A quick way to check this is to look at your urine colour. Ideally you want it to be pale straw in colour. If it is darker, then have a drink! Some of you may also like to drink while you are exercising and this is a useful way to prevent dehydration. Water or no-added-sugar squash should be your preferred choice; remember this is a low-intensity session for no more than 60 minutes with little stress on the body, so the energy demand is also low – there is no need to take on extra fuel. Aim to drink 3–5ml/kg BW of non-nutritive fluid 2 hours before or no more than 200ml/7fl oz every 20 minutes.

A low-intensity training session can be fuelled by converting fat stores to glucose to provide energy for the working muscle; there is no urgency for the muscle to receive energy quickly to maintain a high-intensity level of work. Everybody needs and has fat stores; some may have more than others, but ultimately we all have them and they are there for a reason. They provide energy. Fat is a great fuel for endurance events, but it is simply not adequate for high-intensity exercise such as sprints or intervals. If exercising at a low intensity, you have enough stored fat to fuel activity for hours or even days as long as there is sufficient oxygen to allow fat metabolism to occur.

The emphasis of this book has always been about tailoring your nutrition to your training. In Chapter 1 we looked at how much of each fuel type you need during training. These guidelines tie in directly. For a low-intensity day the recommended carbohydrate intake was 3g/kg BW (see page 15), which shows how little carbohydrate is required when exercising at a low intensity.

EATING TOO MUCH CARBOHYDRATE

What happens if you eat more carbohydrate than you need on these low-intensity training days? It comes back to performance. Most of you have a goal to achieve within your given sport. If you fuel right, you will benefit from your training but you will also help your body to adapt so it becomes more efficient. For some of you this may mean that you lose excess weight, for others it might mean that your body composition (see pages 58–60) changes so that you gain more lean muscle mass. Both of these factors can have a positive influence on your performance. For example, a leaner volleyball athlete will have a higher vertical jump height to ensure clearance of the ball over the net; a lighter, although healthy weight, runner will potentially run faster with fewer pounds to carry!

So by eating more carbohydrate than you need, your body will use this for fuelling this low-intensity session as it converts to glucose a lot quicker and easier than fat. Also remember that the carbohydrate actually needed to fuel this session will be a lot less than when you are working at high intensity. During high-intensity exercise, an individual will use 60g of carbohydrate an hour, the equivalent of one bagel. During low-intensity exercise, this value of carbohydrate will be significantly less, probably around half this value – only 30g in an hour. If you over-consume carbohydrate it will need to be stored within your body, first as glycogen but if these stores are full then as fat. This is not really a problem if it happens occasionally. If, however, you habitually over-consume carbohydrate and store it as fat, you may find that rather than your body adapting to your training, it actually becomes less efficient.

· ·

FOOD AND TRAINING DIARY

When I work with new athletes/clients, I always ask them to complete the following food and training diary for at least 3 days, to build a picture of where an individual is before they start working with me. It is also a helpful tool to demonstrate where changes can be made. You can do this yourself at home to flag up any potential issues and discover where improvements can be made. Record everything you eat and drink and indicate times of food intake, quantity, ingredients of recipes and brands, if not homemade. Also fill in your daily training: times, type and intensity from 1–5, with 1 being an easy session and 5 being a tough session. If possible also try to indicate how you felt during and after your training i.e. tired, energized, sore etc.

Day/Date	Time	Food/Meal	Training/Intensity	Energy indicator
12th November	6.30am		30 mins run – intensity 2-3	Easy, managed a better time than usual
	7am	Toast with peanut butter, smoothie, cup of coffee		
	11am	An apple and a piece of cheese		
	1.30pm	Soup and small brown bread roll		
	5.30pm	A chicken salad and a low-fat yogurt		
	7pm		60-mins intensity 4 training, interval sprints	Lacked energy / not working to full potential

A sample food and training diary for one day

Looking at your chart, you might be able to spot problems with how you are currently fuelling your training. For example, if you tried to do a training session at a high intensity but did not eat appropriate carbohydrate before this, you probably found the session very tough and ran out of energy towards the end. Once you have identified any issues, turn to the meal plans and ensure that you are following an appropriate meal plan for the level of intensity you are training at that day.

CASE STUDY

A few years ago a lady came to see me. She was in her early 40s and had decided to train for a triathlon – just sprint distance, but this was still a big jump from her previous sedentary life. One of her main reasons for taking up exercise was that she wanted to lose weight. She was 6kg (14lb) overweight at this point. She thought that by increasing her training from zero to 4/5 times a week, she would definitely lose weight. However, three months down the line she had seen no change. She felt better in herself and was definitely fitter but she was disappointed and confused that she was not losing weight when she was so much more active than she had been.

From the food and training diary she presented, it was clear that the real issue was that she was not tailoring her nutritional intake to her training or training intensities. So no matter what session she was doing, whether it was a 2-hour BRICK session (bike and then run) or a 30-minute easy swim, she was eating carbohydrate before every session. She was meeting her new energy requirements, which is why her weight stayed the same.

During this initial assessment, we looked at her weekly training and I explained about the different types of training intensity and what this meant nutritionally. I pointed out the sessions where she would definitely need carbohydrate, such as the BRICK, and explained how much she would need and what this looked like practically (see opposite), as well as advising her on how to recover from this session. We also talked about the 'easy' morning swims and how these could actually be done in a fasted state – I explained that this was a really useful way of tapping into fat stores and helping with her weight-loss goals.

I also addressed the importance of portion size – I put a packet of pasta in front of her and asked her to show me how much she usually prepared. I then showed her in weight how much she needed to actually meet her carbohydrate requirement for that meal. She was surprised at how much she had been overeating. This is an example of what she was eating before she came to see me:

Pre-AM training swim (low-intensity session – 45 mins):	2 pieces of toast with jam and butter
During swim:	500ml/17fl oz energy drink
Post-swim:	Porridge/oatmeal made with milk, banana and honey
Lunch:	Chicken and salad sandwich, cereal bar and coffee
Pre-run (moderate-intensity session – 60 mins):	3 pieces of malt loaf
During run:	500ml/17fl oz energy drink
Dinner:	Large helping of spaghetti bolognese, bowl of ice cream

Her carbohydrate requirements for this day were 5g/kg BW and she was actually getting 6.5g/kg BW and a total calorie intake of 2,726. My advice for the same day looked like this:

Swim session:	In fasted state as low intensity and under 60 mins
Post-swim breakfast:	2 pieces of wholemeal toast with 2 boiled/poached eggs
Lunch:	Sweet potato with chicken salad; yogurt and fruit
Pre-pm session:	2 oatcakes with hummus and apple
Post–pm session:	Main meal – stick to $1/2$ plate veg/salads, $1/4$ plate protein and $1/4$ plate carbs, followed by yogurt and fruit
Pm:	Hot chocolate made with milk

This comes in at 5g/kg BW and a total calorie intake of 2,050. We met four weeks later and her weight had decreased from 70kg (154lb) to 67kg (148lb). One of her concerns about changing her eating practices was not having enough energy to train and feeling hungry, but on my plan she felt better. She was still meeting her nutritional needs but her calorie intake was 500–700 less a day, resulting in a steady weight loss over the four weeks. This loss also improved her running times and helped her swim more efficiently.

LOW-INTENSITY TRAINING MEAL PLANS

The following meal plans are ideal for days when you are doing low-intensity exercise, for rest days when you are not exercising at all, or if you are someone who exercises for 3 hours or less a week at any level. They provide the relevant amount of carbohydrate needed, as well as incorporating suitable recovery options.

60 MINUTE LOW-INTENSITY SESSION

Breakfast: Blueberry Bircher Muesli (see page 185)
Lunch: Super Beans on Toast (see page 214); piece of fruit
Snack: Frozen Vanilla Yogurt (see page 280)
Dinner: Baked Seabass with Rice Noodle Salad and Salsa (see page 246); Recovery Hot Chocolate (see page 277)

60 MINUTE LOW-INTENSITY SESSION

Breakfast: Banana and Almond Smoothie (see page 183)
Lunch: Beetroot, Feta and Potato Salad (see page 218)
Snack: Apple and 20g/1 tbsp Nut Butter (see page 191)
Dinner: One-Pot Chicken Casserole (see page 224); Summer Fruit and Mint Kebabs (see page 283)

60-MINUTE LOW-INTENSITY SESSION

Breakfast: Banana and Almond Smoothie (see page 183)
Lunch: Chicken Kebabs with Spiced Tahini (see page 200); Summer Fruit and Mint Kebabs (see page 283) or a fruit salad
Snack: Crudités with Harissa and Cumin Hummus (see page 271)
Dinner: Thai-Style Baked Fish with Stir-Fried Vegetable Rice (see page 244); Summer Fruit and Mint Kebabs (see page 283)

Breakfast: Blueberry Bircher Muesli (see page 185)
60-MINUTE LOW-INTENSITY SESSION
Lunch: Smoked Haddock & Squash Fishcakes (see page 205) with a green salad; milk-based drink such as a latte
Snack: Crudités with Harissa and Cumin Hummus (see page 271)
Dinner: Roasted Vegetable Tortilla Lasagne (see page 255); Fruity Fool (see page 286)

Breakfast: Cranberry and Mango Smoothie (see page 183)
60 MINUTE LOW-INTENSITY SESSION
Lunch: Three-Lentil Dhal with Coriander and Chilli `
     (see page 213);
Snack: 2 oatcakes with Pepper and Yogurt Dip (see page 269)
Dinner: Tangy Chicken Stir-Fry (see page 227); Nectarine
     Compôte with Zesty Crème Fraîche (see page 285)

Breakfast: Summer Fruit Smoothie (see page 182)
Lunch: Chickpea and Kale Broth (see page 211)
Snack: Berry and Toasted Almond Pot (see page 282)
60-MINUTE LOW-INTENSITY SESSION
Dinner: Sausage Casserole (see page 235); Recovery Hot Chocolate
     (see page 277)

Breakfast: Breakfast Shake (see page 182)
Lunch: Prawn and Orange Salad (see page 206)
Snack: 2 Stuffed Dates (see page 275)
60-MINUTE LOW-INTENSITY SESSION
Dinner: Fruity Steak Stir-Fry (see page 233); Frozen Peach Yogurt
     (see page 281)

REST DAY – NO TRAINING
Breakfast: Cinnamon Apple Porridge (see page 187)
Lunch: Courgette and Feta Frittata (see page 208), with a side salad
Snack: Summer Fruit and Mint Kebabs (see page 283)
Dinner: Zesty Mackerel Fillets (see page 243);
     Baked Spiced Apricots (see page 292)

REST DAY – NO TRAINING
Breakfast: Granola Pot (see page 184)
Lunch: Beetroot and Butternut Panzanella (see page 216)
Snack: Fruity Fool (see page 286)
Dinner: Mustard–Mash Chicken Pie (see page 255); piece of fruit

REST DAY – NO TRAINING
Breakfast: Sunflower Seed and Chia Porridge (see page 188)
Lunch: Salmon Chowder (see page 204)
Dinner: Rosemary and Paprika Vegetable and Bean Hot Pot (see
     page 249); Berry and Toasted Almond Pot (see page 282)

MODERATE-INTENSITY TRAINING

This level of training feels like 6/10 RPE or around 60–70 percent of your maximal heart rate. It is the pace at which you feel 'worked'; like the effort you feel when you are walking and suddenly have to climb a hill. You should still be able to have a conversation but it won't feel as easy as when you are doing a low-intensity pace. It should feel like an intensity level that you could train at for up to 90 minutes pain-free and without any additional fuel needs, as it is the pace at which oxygen uptake is still sufficient enough to help clear lactate and pyruvate (see page 56). This pace is also known as 'steady state'.

Determining the exact speed of this pace, whether running, cycling or swimming, will be very individual. For example, for one runner a moderate pace might be 7.45-minute miles and for another it may be more like 8.45-minute miles. For team sports, such as netball or football, moderate-intensity training might be a skills-based session, which involves some drills and game play but is not a session where you finish feeling completely depleted. That is why it is important to think about how you perceive your exertion; although the actual pace may vary slightly from session to session, in physiological terms it will still evoke the same response.

Tip

By working at a moderate-intensity pace, you are continuing to build on your endurance base, while also adapting your body to manage this at a slightly faster pace. For those of you who already have a good aerobic base, this may be the pace at which you do long endurance sessions. Ultimately it is starting to raise the speed you can maintain for longer without causing a sharp increase in lactic acid (see page 55).

In terms of fuelling a moderate-intensity session, to a degree it will depend on how well 'trained' you are. The more comfortable you become working at this pace, the higher percentage of fat you will use. However to start with you will probably find including some carbohydrate prior to exercising at this pace will be of benefit, especially if you plan to train for longer than 60 minutes.

For these types of sessions, it is not essential that glycogen stores are full but having a sensible mix of carbohydrate and protein before heading out will mean that you manage this session more comfortably. I tend to recommend 1g/kg BW carbohydrate and 0.25g/kg of protein the meal before the session.

Here are some good examples of what to include:

For morning sessions:

>>> Scrambled Egg Pitta – see page 192

>>> Breakfast Shake – see page 182

>>> Granola Pot – see page 184

>>> Blueberry Bircher Muesli – see page 185

• •

CAN'T STOMACH FOOD?

I appreciate that some people find it very difficult to stomach any food prior to a training session; it can potentially cause gastro-intestinal upset, leaving you feeling nauseous. Some people get stitch and others just don't like the feeling of fullness. It is recommended that you should eat 1–3 hours prior to training to avoid a stitch. The exact period of time is very individual and you will know what works best for you. If you eat too close to training you may find you develop a stitch, although another common cause of stitches is dehydration.

For those of you who prefer not to eat before training, a moderate-intensity session could be done in a fasted state, especially if you already have a good endurance base. However, in order to benefit from this steady state session, it is important that you distinguish the difference between this pace and your easy pace. This can be difficult to measure in a fasted state, as this slightly faster pace could be perceived as hard without any fuel in the tank!

Those of you with a good endurance base will find that your body is actually more efficient at using fat stores for fuel and so won't find increasing the pace to this intensity as difficult as those of you who are new to the sport. Seasoned athletes still tend to use heart-rate data or other devices such as a watch or app that helps them to ensure they are hitting the correct pace for this moderate-intensity session.

For those of you who do find eating difficult before training but also struggle to hit a moderate-intensity training pace without any carbohydrate in your system, try having a homemade energy drink (see the tip box below) just before you go out or even while you are out.

....

Tip

Try this simple recipe for a homemade energy drink that provides you with 30g of carbohydrate and around 38mmol of sodium total, which is in line with most branded sports drinks: 300ml/10½ fl oz fruit juice, diluted with 200ml/7fl oz water and ¼ teaspoon salt if it is a hot day and you are drinking on the hoof! You might not find the salt palatable first thing if you have not yet sweated!

For those of you who prefer to train later in the day, whether this is around lunchtime, early or even late evening, the key is to include a small amount of carbohydrate in the preceding meals. Again I would recommend around 1g/kg BW carbohydrate at each meal or more simply this usually works out to be about a fist-size portion, as well as your 0.25g protein portion and a good helping of vegetables or salad.

RECOVERING FROM MODERATE-INTENSITY SESSIONS

Remember that this steady state is one that hasn't taxed the body too much so in terms of recovery the window available to refuel will be up to 2 hours of finishing. In most cases this will tie in with your next meal. The only exception to this might be if you choose to train later in the evening when you have already eaten your dinner. You may come home to find you need something to help you recover but also prepare you for bed. The most suitable choice will be dairy-based, as it is easily digestible carbohydrate and protein; the Recovery Hot Chocolate on page 277 was included for this exact scenario. You could also team this with a banana or a piece of toast with nut butter if you feel that the drink alone is not sufficient.

MODERATE-INTENSITY TRAINING MEAL PLANS

Here are sample menus that will work well for moderate-intensity sessions. They have been tailored so that they provide sufficient carbohydrate around your training session as well as suitable recovery options, containing the necessary carbohydrate and protein.

Pre-training: Summer Fruit Smoothie (see page 182)
60-MINUTE MODERATE-INTENSITY SESSION
Breakfast: Sunflower Seed and Chia Porridge (see page 188)
Lunch: Courgette and Feta Frittata (see page 208)
Snack: 2 oatcakes with Harissa and Cumin Hummus (see page 271)
Dinner: Tangy Chicken Stir-Fry (see page 277); Nectarine Compôte with Zesty Crème Fraîche (see page 285)

Breakfast: Cinnamon Apple Porridge (see page 187)
Lunch: Egg Fried Rice with Toasted Cashews (see page 209)
60-MINUTE MODERATE-INTENSITY SESSION
Dinner: Turkey Pesto Kievs (see page 231) with Roasted Mediterranean Vegetables (see page 256); Frozen Peach Yogurt (see page 281)

Pre-training: Nut Butter, Honey and Oat Muffin (see page 190)
60-MINUTE MODERATE-INTENSITY SESSION
Breakfast: Tropical Smoothie (see page 276) with Banana and Nut Butter Sandwich (see page 267)
Lunch: Salmon Chowder (see page 204)
Snack: Milk-based drink such as a latte
Dinner: Half and Half Chilli con Carne (see page 232); Berry and Toasted Almond Pot (see page 282)

Breakfast: Blueberry Bircher Muesli (see page 185)
60-MINUTE MODERATE-INTENSITY SESSION
Post-training: Black Pepper Pitta Crisps (see page 274) with Mackerel Pâté (see page 270)
Snack: Cranberry and Mango Smoothie (see page 183)
Dinner: Punjabi Chicken Biryani (see page 229); Recovery Hot Chocolate (see page 277)

Breakfast: Granola Pot (see page 184)

60 MINS MODERATE-INTENSITY SESSION

Lunch: : Roasted Vegetable and Mozzarella Bruschetta (page 219) and a latte

Snack: Crudités with Harissa and Cumin Hummus (see page 271)

Dinner: Lamb and Spinach Curry (see page 240); Frozen Vanilla Yogurt (see page 280)

30 MINS MODERATE-INTENSITY SESSION

Breakfast: Scrambled Egg Pitta (see page 192)

Lunch: Three-Lentil Dhal with Coriander and Chilli (see page 213)

Snack: Dark Chocolate and Ginger Muffin (see page 260)

30 MINS MODERATE-INTENSITY SESSION

Dinner: Sweet Potato Parcels (see page 254); Summer Fruit and Mint Kebabs (see page 283) or a fruit salad

Breakfast: Breakfast Shake (see page 182)

Lunch: One-Pot Chicken Casserole (see page 224); Poached Pears with Cardamom Custard (see page 293)

2-HOUR MODERATE INTENSITY SESSION

Dinner: Beetroot, Feta and Potato Salad (see page 218); Summer Fruit and Mint Kebabs (see page 283) or a fruit salad

Breakfast: Oaty Banana Pancake (see page 195)

60 MINS MODERATE-INTENSITY SESSION

Lunch: Avocado and Seeded Toast (see page 215)

Snack: Tropical Smoothie (see page 276)

Dinner: Char-grilled Chicken Pasta Salad (see page 230); Berry Meringues (see page 287)

Breakfast: Cinnamon Apple Porridge (see page 187)

Lunch: Beetroot and Butternut Panzanella (see page 216)

Snack: Nut Butter Squares (see page 266)

60 MINS MODERATE-INTENSITY SESSION

Dinner: Coriander Lamb with Quinoa (see page 239); Recovery Hot Chocolate (see page 277)

Pre-training: Summer Fruit Smoothie (see page 182)
60 MINS MODERATE-INTENSITY SESSION
Post training: Granola Pot (see page 184)
Lunch: Tortilla Pizza (see page 207)
Dinner: Roasted Aubergine and Beef Curry (see page 234);
Coconut and Mango Rice Pudding (see page 291)

ENDURANCE TRAINING

Most endurance athletes, so those of you who are training for events that you will complete in over 90 minutes, will do 75 percent of your overall training at low (25 percent) and moderate (50 percent) intensities. This will include at least one if not two longer training sessions, lasting over 90 minutes. These longer endurance sessions are about helping your heart adapt at a cellular level so that you are able to maintain running/swimming/cycling, or all three in the case of an Ironman event, for a long duration, so it is more about 'time training'. Endurance training should put no stress on your body and you should be able to manage a conversation while out doing it; it is not about covering a certain distance in a given time frame but it is about saying, 'Today I am going to go out on my bike for 3 hours!' This helps the body to adapt – for example, it helps cyclists endure sitting in the saddle for long periods or for runners to have time on their feet, providing both physical and psychological preparation.

Nutritionally, these are very interesting sessions to fuel. On the one hand they are at a low to moderate intensity so we know physiologically our fat stores can fuel such sessions for long periods of time. On the other hand, while out training for long hours, especially once you get over the 2-hour mark, there is going to be an energy deficit that needs to be met. So while at this intensity our bodies might only use 30g of glucose per hour, the average female weighing 55kg/121lb will burn in the region of 800 calories in 2 hours – this will vary from individual to individual.

Most of you will probably choose to replace your fuel through carbohydrate choices (see page 18), such as energy gels, jelly babies, energy drinks, cereal bars etc, aiming for your 30–60g of carbohydrate an hour. However these training sessions are also a perfect opportunity to become 'fat adapted' (see overleaf).

FAT ADAPTATION

It has been demonstrated in studies time and time again that both carbohydrate and fat are used as fuel during exercise; the higher the intensity of exercise, the more carbohydrate is utilized as fuel over preference to fat. We have already determined that at lower intensities our fat stores are a valuable source of energy but if we provide our bodies with carbohydrate prior to these low-intensity activities, they will preferentially use this source for fuel as it is in a more readily available form.

In recent years there has been a lot of interest in this concept of becoming 'fat adapted', which simply means that our bodies become trained to use our fat stores even when we are working at a higher intensity. This in turn means that our glycogen stores and carbohydrate fuel source can be spared, resulting in us going faster, therefore working at a higher intensity, for longer during endurance events. Remember that for most of us, full glycogen stores will fuel high-intensity work for up to 90 minutes. The theory suggests that by becoming fat adapted, you can spare these glycogen stores by using more fat stores and prolong the decline in glycogen stores significantly.

Although further research is still needed, many elite athletes are using this technique by 'periodizing' their carbohydrate intake. This means that they still choose to make high-carbohydrate choices around high-intensity training sessions, to ensure that they hit target paces and push their lactate threshold (see page 55). During long endurance training sessions, however, at a low- to moderate-intensity, they avoid carbohydrate before or during to ensure that they only use fat stores to fuel that session.

In practical terms, this means they will have a carbohydrate-free breakfast and then during the session, they will take on fluid, possibly electrolytes if it is very warm but energy calories will be in the form of fat or protein. Holly Rush (GB Marathon Runner and Ultra-runner) swears by salted peanuts – salt, fat and protein but no carbohydrate.

Note: these studies have been done on well-trained athletes so I would not recommend trying this if you are new to endurance sport.

I recommend that you have full glycogen stores prior to these sessions as these will last for 90–120 minutes. Inevitably you are going to run out of glycogen stores – even by topping up with suitable carbohydrate options during the session, you will end up using a mixture of both carbohydrate and fat for fuel.

So how do you ensure you have full glycogen stores? The human body can store around 1,500–2,000 calories worth of carbohydrate as glycogen. For men, this means consuming 500g of carbohydrate in the 24 hours prior to a long endurance training session, and for women 400g. Practically the most important thing is for you to take on sufficient complex carbohydrate at all your meals and snacks. Again this is demonstrated in the meal plans throughout this chapter.

ENDURANCE FUEL

During endurance activity that lasts over 2 hours, every 30–45 minutes aim to consume around 30g of carbohydrate. Some examples are:

>>> A sports gel

>>> 500ml/17fl oz energy drink

>>> 6 jelly babies

>>> 45g/1$\frac{1}{2}$oz raisins

>>> 1 banana

>>> Half a bagel with yeast extract or jam

>>> 2 slices malt loaf

>>> Half a Sweet Potato Brownie (see page 264)

RACE DAY NUTRITION

These long endurance training sessions are also a really good time to practise race-day nutrition, so think about fuelling before, during and after. You will feel more confident on race day if you know that the meals and snacks you have chosen to eat in preparation are tried, tested and unlikely to cause you any tolerance issues. These long training sessions are also a chance to try out energy gels and drinks and sweets that you want to use on race day. Some good meals to choose before a long endurance day include:

>>> Sweet Potato Risotto (see page 250)

>>> Punjabi-Style Aloo Sabsi served with flat bread (see page 252)

>>> Butternut Squash and Coconut Curry with rice (see page 251)

>>> Italian Pasta (see page 257)

These meals have had their protein content exchanged for higher carbohydrate content, in order to help fuel the muscles for the long endurance activity the next day. They make an ideal choice on pre-competition day and so it is a good idea to trial with them before.

RECOVERY FROM ENDURANCE SESSIONS

Recovery from endurance sessions is extremely important. Although you may not have put a huge amount of stress on your cardiovascular system or muscles, you will have completely depleted your glycogen stores. These will need to be replenished as soon as possible.

A combination of carbohydrate and protein is essential as soon as is practically possible: definitely within the first hour of finishing your session and then every 2 hours after that until your next meal. Again, aim for 1–1.2g/kg BW of carbohydrate and 0.25g/kg BW of protein. So let's take a 65kg/143lb male athlete who has been on a 3-hour bike ride, which finished at 2pm. His requirements will be 65–78g carbohydrate and 17g protein:

2.30pm	500ml/17fl oz chocolate milk and banana (75g carbohydrate and 18g protein)
4.30pm	2 slices of wholegrain toast with ½ can baked beans, 150g/5oz fruit yogurt (78g carbohydrate, 17g protein)
6.30pm	3 slices of malt loaf, 50g/1¾oz nuts (any unsalted) (60g carbohydrate, 17g protein)
8.30pm	Main meal

This type of refuelling is even more important if you are planning on a further training session within 24 hours.

ENDURANCE TRAINING MEAL PLANS

Below is a collection of meal plans which take into consideration your requirements for long endurance training sessions. They ensure that you have full glycogen stores prior to training in order to fuel your endurance session, and also include good recovery choices to start rebuilding your glycogen stores as soon as possible.

Breakfast: Race Day Bagel with Nut Butter (see page 191) and Cranberry and Mango Smoothie (see page 183)
ENDURANCE ACTIVITY – FUEL AS REQUIRED
Post-training: Mocha Shake (see page 277)
Lunch: Salmon Muscle-Recovery Wrap (see page 203)

Snack:	Spinach and Parmesan Muffin (see page 272)
Dinner:	Sausage Casserole (see page 235); Greek-Style Potted Lemon Cheesecake (see page 288)
Evening:	Recovery Hot Chocolate (see page 277)
Breakfast:	Buckwheat Pancakes with Strawberries and Vanilla Yogurt (see page 194)
Lunch:	Beef Soba Noodles (see page 201); Dark Chocolate and Ginger Muffin (see page 260)

ENDURANCE ACTIVITY – FUEL AS REQUIRED

Post-training:	Cranberry and Mango Smoothie (see page 183)
Dinner:	Bulgar Wheat Curry (see page 253); Rhubarb Crumble Granola (see page 290)
Evening:	Recovery Hot Chocolate (see page 297) and Banana and Nut Butter Sandwich (see page 267)
Breakfast:	Black Forest Porridge (see page 186)

ENDURANCE ACTIVITY – FUEL AS REQUIRED

Post-training:	Summer Fruit Smoothie (see page 182); Spicy Steak Wrap with Tomato Salsa (see page 202)
Snack:	Latte and slice of Carrot and Ginger Cake (see page 262)
Dinner:	Lamb and Spinach Curry with rice (see page 240); Coconut and Mango Rice Pudding (see page 291)
Breakfast:	2 x Nut Butter, Honey and Oat Muffins (see page 190)
Lunch:	Hearty Vegetable Soup (see page 210) with Cheese and Chilli Scone (see page 273)

ENDURANCE ACTIVITY – FUEL AS REQUIRED

Post-training:	500ml (17fl oz) flavoured milk
Dinner:	Mixed Nut Pesto and Roasted Mediterranean Vegetable Pasta (see page 256); Lemon Drizzle Polenta Cake (see page 289)
Breakfast:	Sunflower Seed and Chia Porridge (see page 188)

ENDURANCE ACTIVITY – FUEL AS REQUIRED

Post-training:	Banana and Almond Smoothie (see page 183) and Chicken Kebabs with Spiced Tahini (see page 200)
Snack:	2 slices Courgette Tea Bread (see page 263) and a latte
Dinner:	Chilli Chard and Pork Rice (see page 236); Poached Pears with Cardamom Custard (see page 293)
Breakfast:	Race Day Bagel with Nut Butter (see page 191)

ENDURANCE ACTIVITY – FUEL AS REQUIRED

Post-training: Root Vegetable Chips with Dippy Eggs (see page 221)
Snack: Mocha Shake (see page 277)
Dinner: Purple Pancetta Penne (see page 237); Frozen Peach Yogurt (see page 281)

Breakfast: Black Forest Porridge (see page 186)
Lunch: Chicken and Quinoa Salad (see page 199)
Snack: Slice of Carrot and Ginger Cake (see page 262)
ENDURANCE ACTIVITY – FUEL AS REQUIRED
Dinner: Scrambled Egg Pitta (see page 192) and Recovery Hot Chocolate (see page 277)

Breakfast: 2 slices Apple Breakfast Bread (see page 189) with honey
ENDURANCE ACTIVITY – FUEL AS REQUIRED
Post-training: Roasted Vegetable and Mozzarella Bruschetta (see page 219) with a milk-based drink
Snack: Cheese and Chilli Scone with chutney (see page 273)
Dinner: Salmon Pasta Bake (see page 245); Frozen Peach Yogurt (see page 281)

Breakfast: Breakfast Shake (see page 182)
Lunch: Avocado and Seeded Toasts (see page 215)
ENDURANCE ACTIVITY – FUEL AS REQUIRED
Post-training: Milk-based drink; oatcakes with Pepper and Yogurt Dip (see page 269)
Dinner: Zesty Mackerel Fillets (see page 243) with quinoa; Lemon Drizzle Polenta Cake (see page 289)

Breakfast: Oaty Banana Pancake (see page 195)
ENDURANCE ACTIVITY – FUEL AS REQUIRED
Post-training: Milk-based drink, Spinach and Parmesan Muffin (see page 272)
Snack: Courgette and Feta Frittata (see page 208)
Dinner: Easy Fish and Chips (see page 247); Greek-Style Potted Lemon Cheesecake (see page 288)

HIGH-INTENSITY TRAINING

This is going to feel like an intensity of 7/10 RPE or above; working at 70 percent or more of your maximal heart rate.

The intensity of your training will depend on your event. So if we say that lactate threshold (see page 55) is 7.5/10, endurance athletes will do their high-intensity training at just under or just over so that they are always working to challenge their lactate threshold. This might be in the form of intervals with equal or slightly less time for recovery at just over their lactate threshold; or a more continuous run for up to 60 minutes just under their lactate threshold. During the 'effort', whether continuous or in intervals, you should be working to a pace where you are unable to say more than a few words. Long-term this should result in a higher lactate threshold, meaning that you will be able to maintain a faster pace before you feel that all too familiar 'burn' and fatigue.

In sprint or team/power sports, these high-intensity sessions are usually done at the very top of the Borg scale (10/10 RPE and at maximum heart rate) so that athletes are really trying to develop their anaerobic system; they usually take the format of maximal short bursts, no more than 30 seconds, with long recovery periods of several minutes. These are all-out efforts so they are extremely hard; you should not be able to say anything and may even get that 'blood in mouth' feeling!

Fuelling these high-intensity sessions is very important but is slightly different depending on whether you are doing an endurance sport or a speed/power sport.

FUELLING FOR THE ENDURANCE ATHLETE

Carbohydrate availability is necessary to achieve a fast pace; the faster you go, the quicker you will use this carbohydrate, up to 60g an hour.

Remember the whole point of these sessions for endurance athletes is to be able to maintain an increased speed for a given distance, such as the case of a marathon. (In ultra-distance events it is unlikely that you will be trying to achieve a faster pace.) It is therefore important that a pace slightly above and slightly below the lactate threshold can be attained. This level of training is demanding of the body and requires a ready supply of carbohydrate – trying to do this type of session on low or empty glycogen stores is not going to be beneficial. You will be unable to achieve a fast pace; you may find you can maintain the pace for the first 10–20 minutes of the session but once your glycogen stores become depleted, your body will have to revert to fat stores to provide energy. We already know that this is a much slower process. This switching from glycogen to fat for fuel is also known as 'bonking' or 'hitting the wall' (see page 56).

If you 'hit the wall', you will feel the immediate shift in speed – you can no longer maintain the faster pace and your body has to slow down; almost like going down a gear in the car when you are going up a hill! If you know you are going out training on low glycogen stores, you can combat this decrease in speed by trying to take on fast-release carbohydrate such as training gels, sweets, dried fruit or sports drinks to keep carbohydrate readily available.

If you know in advance when you are going to do this sort of session, it will help you to organize your nutrition appropriately to ensure you fuel correctly around it. For example, if you are going to do this session on a weekday evening after work, ensure that you have taken on good quantities of complex carbohydrates at breakfast and lunch. As a guideline I would aim for 1g/kg BW carbohydrate at both meals with two snacks of around 0.5g/kg BW carbohydrate. These quantities are, however, a guide and one size does not fit all – so for some of you this may be too much and for others it won't be enough. The key, though, is to ensure that you have taken on carbohydrate regularly leading up to the training session.

HIGH-INTENSITY TRAINING MEAL PLANS

These sample menus will help to show how this all works practically and also demonstrate how to alter your intake depending on what time of day you will be planning on doing the session.

Breakfast:	Cinnamon Apple Porridge (see page 187)
Snack:	Banana and Nut Butter Sandwich (see page 267)
Lunch:	Chicken and Quinoa Salad (see page 199)
Pre-training:	Sweet Potato Brownie (see page 264)

45–60 MINS HIGH-INTENSITY SESSION

Post-training: 250ml/9fl oz flavoured milk

Dinner: Nepalese Chicken with Rice (see page 228);
Berry and Toasted Almond Pot (see page 282)

Evening: Recovery Hot Chocolate (see page 277)

Breakfast: Buckwheat Pancakes with Strawberries and Vanilla
Yogurt (see page 194)

45–60 MINS HIGH-INTENSITY SESSION

Post-training: Tropical Smoothie (see page 276)

Lunch: Salmon Muscle-Recovery Wrap (see page 203);
piece of fruit

Snack: Date Bar (see page 265) and a latte

Dinner: Chicken and Cannellini Stroganoff (see page 226);
Greek-Style Potted Lemon Cheesecake (see page 288)

60 MINS LOW-INTENSITY SESSION

Breakfast: Scrambled Egg Pitta (see page 192)

Pre-training: Banana

45 MINS HIGH-INTENSITY SESSION

Lunch: Sweet Potato and Red Lentil Soup (see page 212); slice
of Lemon Drizzle Polenta Cake (see page 289)

Snack: Cranberry and Mango Smoothie (see page 183)

Dinner: Easy Fish and Chips (see page 247); Mango and Kiwi
Baskets (see page 284); Recovery Hot Chocolate (see
page 277)

Breakfast: Oaty Banana Pancake (see page 195)

Lunch: Roast Sweet Potato and Spinach Wrap with Salsa
(see page 220)

Snack: Slice of Courgette Tea Bread (see page 263)

60 MINS HIGH-INTENSITY SESSION

Post-training: 250ml/9fl oz flavoured milk

Dinner: Moroccan Lamb Stew with couscous (see page 242);
Coconut and Mango Rice Pudding (see page 291)

Evening: Recovery Hot Chocolate (see page 277)

Breakfast: Summer Fruit Smoothie (see page 182)

60 MINS HIGH-INTENSITY SESSION

Post-training: Mocha Shake (see page 277)

Lunch: Root Vegetable Chips with Dippy Eggs (see page 221)

Snack: Banana and Nut Butter Sandwich (see page 267)

Dinner: Bulghır Wheat Curry (see page 253); Frozen Peach Yogurt (see page 281)

Breakfast: Cinnamon Apple Porridge (see page 187)

Lunch: Spicy Steak Wrap with Tomato Salsa (see page 201); slice of Carrot and Ginger Cake (see page 262)

Dinner: Half a serving of Purple Pancetta Penne (see page 237)

60 MINS HIGH-INTENSITY SESSION

Post-training: Recovery Hot Chocolate (see page 277) and Poached Egg Muffins with Avocado (see page 193)

Breakfast: 2 slices Apple Breakfast Bread (see page 189) with Nut Butter (see page 191)

60 MINS HIGH-INTENSITY SESSION

Post-training: Banana and Almond Smoothie (see page 183)

Lunch: Thai Green Chicken Curry (see page 198)

Snack: 2 oatcakes with Pepper and Yogurt Dip (see page 269)

Dinner: Salmon Pasta Bake (see page 245); Baked Spiced Apricots (see page 292)

Breakfast: Blueberry Bircher Muesli (see page 185)

60 MINS HIGH-INTENSITY SESSION

Post-training: 250ml chocolate milk; Date Bar (see page 265)

Lunch: Mushroom, Spinach and Halloumi Salad (see page 217)

Snack: Banana and Nut Butter Sandwich (see page 267)

60 MINS HIGH-INTENSITY SESSION

Post-training: Mocha Shake (see page 277)

Dinner: Sweet and Sour Pork Chops with Sweet Potato (see page 238); Fruity Fool (see page 286)

Breakfast: Buckwheat Pancakes with Strawberries and Vanilla Yogurt (see page 194)

Lunch: Hearty Vegetable Soup (see page 210) with a Cheese and Chilli Scone (see page 273)

Snack: Banana

45 MINS HIGH-INTENSITY SESSION FOLLOWED BY 40-MINS MODERATE-INTENSITY SESSION

Post-training: 250ml (9fl oz) flavoured milk

Dinner: Magic Fish Pie (see page 248); Toasted Rhubarb Granola Crumble (see page 290)

Breakfast: Scrambled Egg Pitta (see page 192)
Lunch: Beef Soba Noodles (see page 201)
Snack: Apple and Walnut Muffin (see page 261)
60 MINS HIGH-INTENSITY SESSION
Dinner: Mushroom and Lamb Moussaka (see page 241);
Coconut and Mango Rice Pudding (see page 291)

FUELLING FOR SPEED/POWER OR TEAM SPORTS

As these high-intensity sessions are working to develop the anaerobic energy system, the actual 'effort' of an all-out interval does not require carbohydrate if the interval is less than 10 seconds. Remember, a maximal effort for less than 10 seconds will be fuelled via the ATP-CP anaerobic pathway (see page 53). If, however, these efforts are longer than 10 seconds but less than 2 minutes, again at maximal effort, they will rely on glycolysis and so require an available source of carbohydrate.

In team sports, it is possible that a high-intensity training session will include drills that involve all out-effort for up to 2 minutes before recovery. Additionally these sessions will last between 1–2 hours, in order to also develop the endurance system of players. So this actually means that carbohydrate requirements will be the same as that of an endurance athlete (see page 85). Practically, then, similar nutritional strategies are useful; planning and ensuring a regular intake of carbohydrate throughout the 24 hours leading up to a high-intensity training session.

RECOVERY FROM HIGH-INTENSITY TRAINING

For all athletes, recovery choices are extremely important after these high-intensity sessions. This may have been a shorter session but due to the intensity at which you have been working, you will have potentially depleted your glycogen stores. This type of session will also have put a lot of stress on your body and so recovery and repair is going to be paramount, especially if you have a further training session within 12 hours, regardless of the type of session ie low intensity, active recovery or weights.

If you have a session within 12 hours, then ensure recovery is within 30 minutes of finishing this session and includes 1.2g/kg BW carbohydrate and 0.25g/kg BW protein in a liquid form with fast-acting carbohydrate and easily digestible protein, eg flavoured milk or a protein and carbohydrate shake.

If it is going to be over 12 hours before your next training session, ensure recovery is within 2 hours of finishing this session and includes 1.2g/kg BW carbohydrate and 0.25g/kg BW protein as a meal, eg a jacket potato with tuna and salad, and a glass of milk.

ACTIVE RECOVERY

This relates to any activity that is done at a low intensity but is different from your normal sport. Most of you will include a rest day or two but some individuals prefer to rest their muscles by doing an activity that works completely different muscles from the ones they tend to use normally. So, for example, if you are a runner, perhaps you will choose to go for a swim; if you are a swimmer, maybe you will go for a jog. A lot of endurance athletes choose activities such as Pilates or yoga that help them with relaxation, stretching and developing core strength.

Whatever activity you choose, it is important to remember that it is a recovery. If you've chosen swimming, it's not about thrashing yourself up and down the pool at the highest intensity possible. This session should complement the rest of your training, allowing your body to rest and recover while still doing an activity.

Nutritionally, there really should be no additional demand on your body for energy or fuel. I tend to count an active recovery day as a rest day. If it falls on the day before an endurance session or a high-intensity training session the following morning, you will need to consider eating enough carbohydrate. However, if it is an isolated day or comes before a low- or moderate-intensity training day, I recommend you keep carbohydrate intake minimal and bulk out meals with vegetables. Continue to include good-quality protein foods, as it is a perfect opportunity for your body to recover and repair itself from hard training earlier in the week.

STRENGTH AND CONDITIONING

So far we have talked about training from a purely speed/endurance perspective. There is another element of training that is now being included regularly in most athletes' training programmes – strength training. Indeed many studies have demonstrated that strength training has real benefits to performance gains.

We know that practising a sport tends to make you better at it, so if you want to get better at running, go running; if you want to get better at football, play football. This type of specific training is very effective up to a point, especially when you are new to a sport. Eventually, though, you will have mastered the techniques to a level where you are able to push your body to its 'natural' limit. So if you are a 200m butterfly swimmer, the natural limit is the point where no matter how much pool practice you do, you cannot improve your personal best time. It is at this point that you may need to 'improve' or 'enhance' your body, both the neuro-muscular (muscle control via the nervous system) and cardiovascular system, as well as looking at the way in which you use your body for your particular sport. The training at different intensities and fuelling we have already looked at help to develop the cardiovascular system. We will now turn our attention to the neuro-muscular system.

Rates of injury can be high in competitive sport. Although participating in sports and exercise is important for good health, sport is not necessarily 'good' for the body from a mechanics and injury point of view. Strength training improves the effectiveness of your ability to practise your sport while preventing injury. Let's consider fast bowlers in cricket: every time they run up to bowl, there is an impact on their lower limbs; there is an imbalance between the right and left side of the body as they bowl repetitively with their dominant arm. Additionally there will be a strain on their spine as they rotate at full speed. Another example is running: you may be familiar with the stresses the impact of the road place on the body if you run outdoors regularly. The next time you are out running, look at the people around you and try to notice differences between the left and right side of their body, as well as the angle of their knees and feet as they make contact with the ground, and the posture of the upper body as they become fatigued. The skeleton is very well designed to distribute load safely, but modern life has caused many of us to develop bad postural habits; our bony frame is limited in the protection it can give us when we have developed poor posture and bad alignment in that our body is no longer 'stacked up' and 'balanced'. This will cause a stress or strain somewhere in the system when we place stress on it during sport, and if we are not aware of this, and do not address it, an overuse injury is inevitable (see Chapter 4).

This section will introduce a variety of training methods and modes that can be used alongside sport-specific training to improve posture, movement and technique, which may reduce the risk of injury and will result in improved performance.

Here are some terms that are often used to describe types of strength and conditioning training:

>>> Strength training

>>> Stability training

>>> Speed training

>>> Body composition gains

>>> Endurance and conditioning

The terminology in the fitness and strength training industries can be very confusing so this section will attempt to describe the key principles behind physical training and link this to practical examples while underpinning scientific theory. The aim of this section is for you to be able to choose the appropriate training methods and nutrition strategy that will balance your overall programme and help you to achieve your performance goals.

Before we move, let's remind ourselves that training means to undertake a physical activity that causes the body to adapt. Your goal or desired training effect is a description of the adaptation you are aiming for, whether that is to:

>>> Increase muscle size

>>> Jump higher

>>> Run faster

>>> Improve body composition (see page 58)

To achieve this adaptation, you must provide the correct training stimulus to the body.

STRENGTH TRAINING

The term 'strength' in a training context can be used to describe the amount of force our muscles can produce or resist, often related to how much extra load we can lift, pull or push. We shouldn't just think about a weight-training analogy to describe strength. Strength or the application of force is essential to all movement and sport. It is a general misconception that sports where you do not lift weights do not need strength. Many such examples exist:

••

OVERLOAD

The training principle of 'overload' involves providing a sufficient training stimulus to the body that is more than the 'normal' training load. So, for example, if you find jogging 5km is a breeze and you practise jogging 5km repeatedly without increasing your distance or speed, your body will cease to continue adapting to this training – the training has become normal and the body can cope without having to adapt. This is a situation where the training stimulus is not sufficient to cause overload.

To cause an overload, you will need to increase the speed or the distance of your run. This will increase the capacity of your heart and lungs to provide energy to the muscles for the new speed or distance; you may also change the shape, size and function of the leg muscles to cope with the greater impact and force produced from each stride.

That said, the human system is not that simple and adaptation often occurs after the training has finished as various hormones are released causing the body to react to the training. Nutrition and rest will have a huge part to play in this adaptation process; if you do not rest your body sufficiently after training or provide it with the necessary fuel it needs at the right time, adaptation to your training will be affected.

••

>>> When we jump, we use our leg muscles to bend and straighten the joints of the lower limb to *push* into the floor as hard and as fast as possible to get maximum jump height – this is a critical movement for netball, volleyball, badminton and many other sports.

>>> When we run, we *push* into the floor in an 'up and down' fashion and also back against the floor in a 'backward and forward' fashion in order to move forward without falling over – so to run faster we need to *push* harder or more often.

>>> When we paddle a kayak, we *pull* on the blade in the water while *resisting* rotation with our core muscles. So how does this relate to the training of strength?

Most of us reach a point when we are unable to produce the force required for the task at hand and this is when we look to strength training to improve. For example, if you need to jump 50cm/20in to compete against an opponent on a volleyball court but your leg strength only allows you to produce a big enough *push* to jump 30cm/12in, you need to adapt your leg muscles using strength training. If you can jump 50cm/20in but your jump is too slow compared with your opponent, then you need to adapt your nervous system to *push* faster.

There are many adaptations that can occur with strength training to increase the amount of force your muscles can produce, or to produce it quicker and more effectively. The easiest to understand is 'hypertrophy'. This is an increase in the size of the cross-sectional area of the muscle fibres. A bigger muscle can produce more force, or a bigger push; think of flicking an elastic band, a bigger elastic band will go further than a small one when stretched to its limit and then released – the principle is similar. Another way to understand this using our running example is to imagine the leg muscles as springs; every time you contact the floor, the spring will compress and then return to its full length, propelling you forward – a bigger spring will have a better result than a small spring.

Your body composition (see page 58) will have a part to play here. The spring will have a greater effect on a lighter body than a heavy body, or a heavy body will require a bigger spring for the same effect. That is why reducing body fat is important for optimal sport performance; extra load or 'dead weight' being carried by the muscles will reduce the effectiveness of our pulls and pushes.

However, doesn't increasing muscle size increase body weight? In some sports muscle can be considered a useful weight as it increases force but in sports where we need to overcome our body weight, such as gymnastics or endurance running, there is a balance to strike. The good news is that we can increase our strength, or amount of push by changing how our nervous system and brain use the muscle fibres effectively without necessarily making sustained excessive increases in muscle size. We can also increase the effectiveness of our tendons, which attach the muscles to the bones.

MAXIMAL STRENGTH TRAINING

In Chapter 1 we looked at muscle type and how having a higher proportion of fast-twitch muscle fibres can generate a lot more force in a short period of time. In order to recruit these fast-twitch fibres in particular, we must use the correct training stimulus, such as a heavy weight, that can only be lifted a few times with maximal effort. This is known as 'maximal strength training' and requires significant skill and practice to be done safely and effectively. Those of us who are fairly new to weight-training, or who do not want to

Tip *Make sure you are training the muscles and tendons that are useful for your sport, not just the ones that make us look good; bigger biceps do not often equal better football!*

risk injury from lifting very heavy weights, can still use this method using a 'fairly heavy' weight that can only be lifted 5–6 times with good technique and near maximum effort. This type of training will usually cause a combination of improvement to the nervous system plus small gains in muscle size. The key is the intent to lift near maximum – this causes the brain to recruit the biggest and fastest muscle fibres.

FUELLING STRENGTH TRAINING

Strength training usually occurs alongside other training and so there are no specific meal plans for this section. However, protein pulsing (see page 26) is the best method of ensuring that your muscles have a constant supply of amino acids to enhance recovery and repair. This is particularly important around these maximal strength-training sessions. Aim to include 0.25g/kg BW of protein 45–60 minutes before and also within 1–2 hours of finishing your session.

Ideally take protein in the form of foods that are high in branched-chain amino acids (see below) such as meat, dairy foods and legumes before a session and then a liquid form of protein, which is easily digestible, after such as milk or whey protein.

So for 70kg/154lb, athletes this would be 18g of protein before and after which in practical terms would be:

>>> 1 hour before maximum strength training: 100g/3½oz chicken

>>> 1–2 hours post-training: 500ml/17fl oz skimmed milk

TARGET NUTRITION

Branched-chain amino acids are essential nutrients that the body obtains from proteins found in food, especially meat, dairy products and legumes, and they include leucine, isoleucine, and valine. 'Branched-chain' refers to the chemical structure of these amino acids. Athletes use branched-chain amino acids to improve exercise performance and reduce protein and muscle breakdown during intense exercise.

EXPLOSIVE STRENGTH TRAINING

To increase the speed of the nervous system signal (ie to jump faster), we may use explosive strength training to use the muscle fibres faster. This type of training involves improving the speed or frequency of the signals from the brain to the muscle and preparing other tissues, such as tendons, to cope with high-speed movements:

>>> Ballistic weight-lifting – using momentum and very intensive pushes and pulls during certain types or weight-lifting such as a 'power clean', when you lift a weight clear above your head

>>> Normal range of lifts but with a lighter weight and attempting to perform the correct movement as fast as possible

One method to improve the 'stiffness' of the tendons to transfer the force produced by the muscle is plyometrics. From a training perspective this includes hopping, and bounding and rebound jumping.

Although the training types described here look like different training sessions, most athletes will do a combination and are likely to emphasize one or the other depending upon the demands of the sport and their stage of development or the time of year. Remember, shot-putters and gymnasts both need to be strong but require differences in body mass and type of strength to perform optimally, so they will have very different 'strength' programmes. Tennis players, rugby players and many other sports may require a mixture of methods to optimize performance.

TARGET TRAINING

The key to power and plyometrics training is the intent to move as fast as possible. Why do you need to train the body to produce force quickly? The reason is often defined by the sport itself – say it takes 1 second to produce your maximal force but when you run or change direction your foot is only in contact with the ground for one-fifth of a second, the more of your force that you can produce in the time frame the sport has given you, the more effective you will be.

Summary

>>> Training is essential for boosting your performance, but different types of training have different nutritional requirements

>>> Training will vary between endurance, sprint/power and team sports, and it's important to exercise the correct energy system required for your sport

>>> Gauging the intensity of your exercise (by using the Borg Scale to obtain your perceived level of exertion) is important in knowing which fuel is best

>>> Your training week will include a mixture of low/rest, moderate and high-intensity training days, which each have an appropriate meal plan, shaped around fuelling and recovering from that level of intensity

>>> There is a variety of strength and conditioning methods that will help to minimize the likelihood of injury, and will help to improve your performance beyond what you can achieve by practising that sport alone

CHAPTER 3:
WHAT'S YOUR SPORT?

FOCUSING ON YOUR DISCIPLINE

In the opening chapters of this book, I talked about how the road to performance gains is a collaborative journey. So far we have looked at the major nutrients, how your body works when you exercise and how this translates into a fuelling strategy. However, some of you may still be questioning how this all fits in with your specific sport and your chosen discipline or distance within that sport.

In this chapter you can take what you have read so far and apply that knowledge to your particular sport by flicking straight to that section (you don't need to read the parts on the sports that you don't practise). We will look at training sessions, nutritional demands and how this all works with your lifestyle.

RUNNING

As I mentioned in the previous chapter, regardless of whether you are training for a 5K, 10K, half marathon, marathon or longer, your training plan will include a variety of training sessions spanning low-, medium- and high-intensity training. The number of each of these sessions will depend a little on the distance you are doing and how many days a week you want to train. The table overleaf is just an example – always ensure you follow a training plan devised by a qualified coach/running website to avoid injury or over-training and work the correct energy systems for your chosen distance. If you are training for a marathon, there is no benefit in running short intervals of around 30 seconds, as this will work and enhance the wrong energy system. Think back to Chapter 1 where we looked at energy systems. When training for a marathon it is beneficial to do intervals, but they need to be longer, around 3–5 minutes. Short intervals work the anaerobic system whereas longer intervals use the aerobic system and it is this system that needs to be pushed so that you can start to improve your lactate threshold. By improving your lactate threshold you will be able to run at a faster pace for a longer period of time before the build-up of lactate becomes limiting to your performance.

Similarly, if you are a 5K runner there is no benefit in doing an endurance run of over 90 minutes as, although it will build overall aerobic fitness, it is not going to sharpen your speed. In fact, it will probably cause additional fatigue because you are likely to be too tired to get the most out of your other sessions.

Some of you may like to include some strength work (see page 99) during the week. Depending on the strength training involved, I would suggest either trying to fit it in between hard training days or maybe even on the same day as a low-intensity session.

Distance	Number of low-intensity/recovery runs per week	Number of low- to moderate-intensity endurance runs over 90 minutes per week	Number of moderate-intensity/steady runs per week	Number of high-intensity/intervals or tempo runs per week	Rest/active rest days per week
5k	1	0	1–2	2–3	1–3
10K	1	0	2	2–3	1–2
Half marathon	1	1	2	2	1
Marathon	1	2 with one containing more specific race pace work	1	2	1
Ultra-marathon	0	3	1	1–2	1–2

TABLE 3.1 An example of a weekly training schedule

Before we go into the specifics of actual training sessions, let's think back to your goal. Most of you, whatever distance you are going to run, are likely to have some sort of time goal in mind, whether that is a 4-hour marathon or a 20-minute 5K. These times are likely to be dictated by previous attempts. You will also be aware that you will need to run at a certain pace to achieve that time goal.

So, for example, to complete a 5K in 20 minutes you will need to be running a 6.26-min/mile pace; at this distance, this will be 20–25 seconds faster than your lactate threshold. By knowing this, it makes it easier to work out what pace your other training sessions should be; intervals will be run at this pace or slightly faster still but moderate-intensity runs will be 30–40 seconds slower. Remember, though, to be realistic – use previous experience to work out what is achievable.

Let's look at some examples of actual training sessions in relation to what they look like, feel like and what nutritional demands they might have.

LOW-INTENSITY TRAINING

Regardless of what distance you are training for, a low-intensity run will always follow the same format: it will be a maximum of 60 minutes run at an easy pace – around 50 percent of your maximum heart rate. While running at this pace, you should be able to have a conversation. It is run between 90 seconds to 2 minutes slower than your race pace; it can be slower but not quicker and you will feel more energized after this type of run, making it useful to put in between two harder sessions.

FUEL REQUIREMENTS

A low-intensity, easy-pace run has no fuel demands. It can be done at any time that works for you but there is no need for any specific fuelling strategy in preparation. So on a day that you are doing one of these runs, your maximum carbohydrate requirements are 3g/kg BW and your protein requirements will be 3–4 servings of 0.25g/kg BW a day. This can be easily achieved by sticking to three meals a day, combining fist-size portions of complex carbohydrate foods, such as oats, sweet potato, root vegetables or pulses with a palm-size portion of protein such as eggs, chicken or fish, served with unlimited undressed salad or vegetables. Snack on fruit or vegetables.

> **Tip** *A great time to do these easy paced runs is first thing in the morning in a fasted state as your body will obtain what it needs from your fat or glycogen stores.*

Take some time to refer back to the low-intensity training sample menus in Chapter 2 (see page 76). These are really helpful in demonstrating how to meet the nutritional requirements for a low-intensity training and rest days. They incorporate recipes from this book, which are suitable to serve up to the whole family while still making sure you're meeting your training needs.

MODERATE-INTENSITY TRAINING

These moderate-intensity runs will look a little different depending on your distance goal. Some training scenarios might include:

FOR A 5K, 10K OR A HALF MARATHON

Some of your moderate-intensity training sessions will be 'tempo' runs. These sessions take the format of a 10-minute warm up, immediately followed by 20–40 minutes at a faster pace about 30 seconds slower than your race pace and close to your lactate threshold. This tempo pace will feel hard but controlled; you won't be able to talk comfortably but it should not feel as if you're racing.

FOR A MARATHON

You will include 'steady state runs'. Marathon runners have a race pace set 20–30 seconds below their threshold pace. Remember your lactate threshold is the pace you can hold for 30–60 minutes (the better trained you are, the longer you will be able to hold this lactate threshold) before the acidity levels become too high in the muscle and you need to stop or slow down. A marathon is going to take longer than an hour, which is why the race pace for a marathon is set slightly slower than your lactate threshold. These 'steady state' moderate-intensity runs will be 30–40 seconds below your race pace and 60 seconds slower than your threshold pace. This pace will feel controlled with some effort but should not feel hard.

FOR ALL DISTANCES, INCLUDING ULTRA DISTANCE

This moderate-intensity training will be a 60–90-minute undulating run where you will run easy on the flats but work harder on the hills, making the overall feel for this run a moderate intensity.

FUEL REQUIREMENTS

This session is harder than an easy run but you are still running within your comfort zone. Your daily carbohydrate requirement will be a maximum of 5g/kg BW and your protein requirement will be 0.25g/kg BW four times a day. The moderate-intensity sample menu plans in Chapter 2 demonstrate what these requirements look like practically and also take into account the time of day you do your run.

If you are an experienced runner, you may feel confident doing this moderate-intensity session early in the morning in a fasted state but do ensure you are hydrated and keep the session to a maximum of 60 minutes. If, however, this session is going to be 60–90 minutes or is scheduled for the day after a hard training session, you will need to have some fuel before your run. Some good examples include:

>>> Banana

>>> 1–2 pieces of malt loaf

>>> 1 piece of toast

>>> Small pot of fat-free Greek yogurt with 1–2 tsp honey

Take time to think about your recovery needs after your run (see page 51). Aim for 1g/kg BW carbohydrate and 0.25g/kg BW protein and also bear in mind the time frame.

If this is your only training session for the day, aim to eat your recovery meal or snack within two hours of completing your run. For most of you this will fall at your next meal. For example, you go out for a steady state run before breakfast at 6.30am and return at 7.30am. You are not planning to do any further training today. The key is to have a good recovery breakfast option, such as Blueberry Bircher Muesli (see page 185) or Scrambled Egg Pitta (see page 192) by 9.30am. It's your choice if you want to have this as you walk back through the door or if you would prefer to have a shower first!

If you are planning to do a second training session within the next 12 hours and your next meal is not imminent after this run, you will need a recovery choice such as the Tropical Smoothie (see page 276) within 30 minutes followed by a meal two hours later.

ENDURANCE TRAINING

These are all runs over 90 minutes. They are relevant to anyone training for a half-marathon distance or more. Three example scenarios are:

1. **2-hour run at an easy to moderate pace, so around 60–90 seconds slower than your half marathon or marathon pace. You should be able to maintain this pace evenly for the whole duration while still managing a conversation.**

2. **2-hour run plus an off-road undulating run, where the pace continually changes with the terrain.**

3. **2–3 hour run at an easy pace, 2 minutes slower than your race pace with a middle section of 4–6 miles run at race pace, finishing with an easy pace.**

Nutritionally these endurance runs are demanding as glycogen stores will be depleted. You will need to prepare 24 hours prior to these runs, taking on sufficient amounts of carbohydrate beforehand, as well as during the run.

FUEL REQUIREMENTS

The key nutrition strategy here is to consume small amounts of carbohydrate in the 24 hours before your training run at every meal and snack. As a rule of thumb, stick to a fist-size portion of a complex carbohydrate choice, 4–6 times during the day. Visually this will look like:

>>> 50g/1¾oz rolled oats

>>> Banana

>>> Fist-size portion of sweet potato

>>> 3–4 oatcakes

>>> Fist-size portion of cooked rice/couscous

>>> Piece of toast

This little and often approach is important as it allows for more efficient glycogen storage and causes less stomach discomfort or problems during your long run. Getting into the habit of this fuelling strategy will be beneficial for race day too. Have a look at the endurance training sample menus in Chapter 2 to become more familiar with this type of fuelling. Once you've sorted your pre-training nutrition, it is time to think about what you might need during your run. This will depend on what sort of long training run it is.

So if you are doing a long off-road trail run, as in scenario 2 above, you might prefer to take a variety of snacks alternating between fast-release options, such as energy bars, and real-food options such as salted peanuts. With these types of runs, it is about getting the balance right between energy requirements and nutrient requirements. What do I mean by this? Remember these runs are not high intensity so they don't need carbohydrate as an available fuel source; by using the fuelling strategy described earlier in this section, you will have full glycogen stores. These full stores will provide you with fuel for around 90 minutes to 2 hours at a low-moderate intensity pace. Once this has been used up, your body will switch to fat stores within the body to enable you to keep running. As carbohydrate is not a necessary fuel in these situations, I always advise that individuals should choose foods/snacks that they will want to eat en route. When you are out running for this length of time, it becomes a mental challenge as well as a physical one and if you have little treats/snacks that you are looking forward to eating, you are more likely to complete your run successfully. I know a lot of ultra-runners who would choose a pork pie over a handful of jelly babies!

Tip *During an endurance run, aim to eat a handful of jelly babies (5–6), half a yeast extract sandwich or three dates every 45 minutes after the first hour.*

If your endurance run is scenario 1 or 3, then it will be better for you to stick with whatever fuel you are considering using in your actual race. This might be energy drinks, energy gels or jelly babies, or a mix of all three.

Remember that during higher-intensity exercise you will use around 60g of carbohydrate an hour, but in these more leisurely paced training sessions you will need half that much.

Aim for one of the following every 45 minutes of training, after your first hour:

>>> 1 gel

>>> 4–5 jelly babies

>>> 500ml/17fl oz energy drink

So if you are going out for a 3-hour run at an easy pace, you will need two gels.

If you are doing a session with race pace in the middle, take one of your gels a mile before. For example, if miles 6–12 are going to be at race pace, take your gel at mile 5. This will ensure that there is carbohydrate available to maintain this higher-intensity pace.

HIGH-INTENSITY TRAINING

These training sessions are going to be done very close to or above your lactate threshold. Remember, the key to these sessions is to improve your lactate threshold, meaning that you will be able to run at a faster speed for longer before it becomes too difficult to maintain due to acid build-up. Here are three training scenarios, based on your distance goal:

1. **For those of you training for distances up to 10K, a typical high-intensity session will be four sets of 4 x 400m with a 1-minute recovery between each repetition and 3 minutes between each set. This is going to feel difficult; you will be breathing very hard as your body will be attempting to consume enough oxygen to prevent the build-up of acid. The 3 minutes between sets will also help to allow some buffering but this session will leave you feeling very depleted and fatigued.**

2. **For a half marathon or marathon, you will work closer to your threshold pace at longer intervals; 6 x 6 minutes with 2 minutes recovery between each 6-minute effort. As each effort is 6 minutes, you will be challenging your lactate threshold, breathing hard but controlled so that you can keep this pace for the 6 minutes. If you start these efforts too hard, you will struggle to keep a constant pace over the six efforts. By repeating this session week after week, the aim will be that eventually these 6-minute efforts will be run at a faster pace, meaning that you have increased your lactate threshold.**

3. **For off-road or ultra distance runs, a typical session will include long hill repetitions. For example, 10 x 4-minute hills then a jog down. Again the key is to build on speed, power and strength, so aiming to keep the time it takes to do your first repetitions consistent throughout all 10 repetitions.**

FUEL REQUIREMENTS

These high-intensity training sessions need carbohydrate. You will be unable to do this type of session without it in your system. Your daily requirements of carbohydrate will be as high as 5g/kg BW in females and 7g/kg BW in males. This equates to 5–7 fist-size portions of carbohydrate distributed throughout the day as meals and snacks. You will also need 4–6 palm-size portions or 0.25g/kg BW protein.

If you are planning to do this training session in the morning, pay attention to consuming carbohydrate in your main meal the night before. Aim for 1–2g/kg BW as a serving size. Follow this up with a similar portion at breakfast at least 1–2 hours before you plan to train.

If you are planning to do this type of session in the evening, ensure you consume 1g/kg BW carbohydrate at breakfast, lunch and a pre-training snack prior to the session.

Have a look at the high-intensity sample menus in Chapter 2 to see how you can ensure you meet your fuel needs depending on when you are training.

After such a hard session, recovery is going to be important. If you have a session within 12 hours, ensure recovery is within 30 minutes of finishing the session and includes 1.2g/kg BW carbohydrate and 0.25g/kg BW protein in a liquid form with fast-acting carbohydrate and easily digestible protein. A good option is flavoured milk or a Mocha Shake (see page 277).

If your next training session is over 12 hours, ensure recovery is within 2 hours of finishing this session and includes 1.2g/kg BW carbohydrate and 0.25g/kg BW protein as a meal. Try Bulgar Wheat Curry (see page 253).

PLANNING YOUR TRAINING WEEK

Although it is important to fuel each training day according to the type of session, you also need to think about how this all flows together in a week. So let's look at the marathon training schedule as an example (see table, below): Monday, Wednesday and Saturday are low-intensity days, so your body doesn't require carbohydrate for energy. However, each one is before a day you are going to do a high-intensity or endurance run, which means sufficient carbohydrate must be eaten in preparation. The easiest way to do this would be to have a carbohydrate-based meal on Monday and Wednesday evening. Similarly, you should aim to eat small regular amounts of carbohydrate throughout Saturday, ready for Sunday.

Monday	Tuesday	Wednesday	Thursday	Friday	Saturday	Sunday
Easy 5-mile run, no more than 60 mins	Track session or long intervals – 60–90 mins	Rest or active recovery (low-intensity) i.e. swimming 30 mins / yoga 60 mins	Marathon race pace session (60–90 mins)	Steady run (60 mins)	Rest	Long run (90 mins– 4 hours)

TABLE 3.2 A weekly training schedule for a marathon

CHANGING DISTANCES

Another area that can be challenging and confusing is moving up in distance from half marathon or less to long training runs for a marathon distance. Many people find it difficult to get the balance right and often over-consume carbohydrate, resulting in weight gain while they are training for their first marathon. Others underestimate their nutritional needs and don't consume sufficient carbohydrate, resulting in them struggling to complete training runs or becoming injured.

CASE STUDY

One of my clients was a 38-year-old mum of two who was stepping up from a half marathon distance to full marathon. Her half marathon PB was 1 hour 49 and she was hoping to complete the Nice marathon toward the end of the year in around 4 hours.

She came to see me because since stepping up her mileage for marathon training, she had been feeling low in energy, especially during high-intensity sessions. She also found that she was having really intense sugar cravings mid-afternoon and succumbing to the biscuit barrel/cookie jar on a regular basis during the week.

An example day was as follows:

6.30am	1 slice wholemeal toast with peanut butter; half grapefruit
8am	60 mins high-intensity intervals (*she reported that she had felt very sluggish at the start of the session and very tired after*)
9.45am	Cup of coffee with semi-skimmed milk (*she reported low energy and blood-sugar but chose not to eat anything*)
11am	1 slice wholemeal toast with half a can of tuna
3pm	2 oatcakes with almond butter, 4 squares of chocolate and a mug of low-calorie hot chocolate
5.30pm	half a chicken breast with some green beans
7pm	1 scoop of ice cream, 1 small banana and a baked apple

She was also worried about over-consuming carbohydrate, as she did not want to gain weight. I went through her sample diet and explained that because she had not consumed sufficient carbohydrate around her high-intensity training, it was leaving her body depleted and that is why she was craving sugar toward the afternoon. Not eating enough complex carbohydrate, which would release energy slowly throughout the day, was actually resulting in her over-consuming the fast-release high-sugar options such as chocolate and ice cream, causing further fluctuations in blood sugar, leaving her low in energy.

I provided her with advice and a nutrition plan that matched her training needs by decreasing carbohydrate around her low-intensity sessions and increasing protein to help her feel full. I recommended she had more carbohydrate prior to and after high-intensity sessions. I suggested that she limited sweet/fast-release carbohydrates to after training to help with blood-sugar control. I also advised on portion sizes of carbohydrate, protein and provided her with recipes she could use for the whole family. Here is an example menu:

Pre-morning high-intensity session: 50g/1¾ oz rolled oats with banana and honey/peanut butter

Post-morning session – recovery choice such as 250ml/9fl oz flavoured milk and a banana

Lunch – protein choice and unlimited salad/veg (I provided her with a list of non-carbohydrate meals)

Mid-afternoon snack – As this was her worst time of day I suggested she choose from the 20g protein list (see page 26) to help with satiety. Good options include fat-free Greek yogurt with stewed blueberries; cottage cheese with carrots; banana with peanut butter through the middle; an apple with 8–10 Brazil nuts; another 250ml/9fl oz carton chocolate milk or a fruit and yogurt smoothie – I provided her with a sheet of ideas.

Dinner – see meal choices with carbohydrates

Evening – a dairy option such as fat-free Greek yogurt with some fruit or hot chocolate made with skimmed milk

I met up with her again six weeks later and she told me that she was feeling much better; she was no longer raiding the biscuit barrel/cookie jar or stopping off to buy a chocolate bar at the petrol station. She had not gained weight and she was on target with her marathon training.

CYCLING

The participation in cycling events has increased significantly over the last few years; the London Olympic legacy has meant a record number of cycling events being launched and attended.

Cycling sportive can take the format of single-day races ranging in distances from a few kilometres up to several hundred kilometres, such as time trials or the London to Brighton Bike Ride. Or they can be multi-stage events, such as the Tour de France or the Cape Epic Mountain Bike Stage Race, covering huge distances over several days.

All cycling primarily requires strength and endurance, although anaerobic capacity is also important for breakaways, hill climbing and all-out sprints to the line. A good training plan will include sessions that will challenge all aspects of these requirements, as shown in the table below:

Day of the week	Training intensity
Monday	60 mins high intensity
Tuesday	60 mins low intensity, recovery ride building on aerobic base
Wednesday	Rest or strength training
Thursday	80 mins high intensity
Friday	90-mins moderate intensity bike ride keeping a constant pace
Saturday	Rest or strength training
Sunday	3-hours plus low–moderate intensity endurance ride

TABLE 3.3 A typical week of cycling training

Depending on the event they are training for, elite athletes will aim to cover in the region of 400–800km (250–500 miles) a week during peak training.

Serious recreational riders, like those of you who are reading this book, will aim to cover around 240–320km (150–200 miles) a week when training for a specific event. With this in mind, nutritional strategies are going to be imperative, especially if you are juggling your training with working and family life. So let's look at some examples of actual training and their nutritional demands.

LOW-INTENSITY TRAINING

Regardless of the distance you are training for, a low-intensity recovery bike ride will always take the same format. It will be a maximum of 60 minutes at an easy pace at around 50 percent of your maximal heart rate, and it will build on your overall aerobic endurance. At this pace you can ride easily while also having a conversation. You will feel more energized after this type of ride, making it useful to put in between two harder sessions.

FUEL REQUIREMENTS

A low-intensity, easy-pace ride has no fuel demands as long as it is kept to a maximum of 60 minutes. A great time to do these easy-paced rides is first thing in the morning in a fasted state, as your body will obtain what it needs from your fat or glycogen stores. That said, these easy-pace rides can be done at any time that works for you but there is no need for any specific fuelling strategy in preparation.

So on a day when you are doing an easy-pace, low-intensity training ride, your maximum carbohydrate requirement is 3g/kg BW and your protein requirement will be 3–4 servings of 0.25g/kg BW a day. This can be easily achieved by sticking to three meals a day, combining fist-size portions of complex carbohydrate foods such as oats, sweet potato, root vegetables or pulses with a palm-size portion of protein such as eggs, chicken or fish, served with unlimited undressed salad or vegetables. Snack on fruit or vegetables.

Take some time to refer back to the low-intensity sample menus in Chapter 2. These are really helpful in demonstrating how to meet the nutritional requirements for low-intensity training and rest days. They incorporate recipes from this book, which are suitable to serve up to the whole family while still making sure you're meeting your training needs.

MODERATE-INTENSITY TRAINING

Moderate-intensity training rides are usually 'steady state', varying in time from 60–90 minutes. This is faster than your 'easy' pace. You should be able to carry on a conversation but may have to occasionally take an extra breath between sentences. If you use a heart-rate monitor, it will be working at around 60–70 percent of your maximal heart rate.

These sessions can be done on the road, or on a turbo trainer or spinning bike but remember to keep to the right intensity.

FUEL REQUIREMENTS

This session is harder than an easy ride but you are still cycling within your comfort zone. Your daily carbohydrate requirement will be a maximum of 5g/kg BW and your protein requirement will be 0.25g/kg BW four times a day. The moderate-intensity sample menu plans in Chapter 2 demonstrate what these requirements look like in real terms, and also take into account the time of day you ride.

If you are an experienced cyclist, you may feel confident doing this moderate-intensity session early in the morning in a fasted state, but do ensure you are hydrated and keep the session to a maximum of 60 minutes. If this session is going to be 60–90 minutes or is scheduled for the day after a hard training session, you will need to have some fuel before your ride. Some good examples include:

>>> Banana

>>> 1–2 pieces of malt loaf

>>> Piece of toast

>>> Small pot of fat-free Greek yogurt with 1–2 tsp honey

Take time to think about your recovery needs after your ride. Aim for 1g/kg BW carbohydrate and 0.25g/kg BW protein and also bear in mind the time frame.

If this is your only training session for the day, aim to eat this recovery meal or snack within 2 hours of completing your ride. For most of you this will fall at your next meal. For example, you go out for a steady state ride before breakfast at 6.30am and return at 7.30am. You are not planning on doing any further training today. The key is to have a good recovery breakfast, such as Blueberry Bircher Muesli (see page 185) or Scrambled Egg Pitta (see page 192) by 9.30am. It's your choice if you want to have this as you walk back through the door or if you would prefer to have a shower first!

If you are planning on a second training session within the next 12 hours, and your next meal is not imminent after this ride, you will need a recovery choice such as the Tropical Smoothie (see page 276) within 30 minutes, followed by a meal 2 hours later.

ENDURANCE TRAINING

The endurance ride is fundamental to any of you who are preparing for a whole-day or multi-day event. It will build in the length of time you are in the saddle as the weeks of training progress. These rides are developing your endurance and aerobic fitness; they should be done at an easy to moderate pace. You should be able to carry on a conversation during a long ride – if you cannot, you are working your body too hard!

Some example scenarios include:

>>> 3.5-hour ride at an easy pace with a fast finish

>>> 4-hour ride over a hilly route

>>> 5-hour ride at an easy pace with a fast finish

Nutritionally these endurance rides are demanding and glycogen stores will be depleted. You will need to prepare 24 hours prior to this, taking on sufficient amounts of carbohydrate before as well as during the training session.

FUEL REQUIREMENTS
The key nutrition strategy for endurance training is to consume small amounts of carbohydrate in the 24 hours before your cycling session at every meal and snack. You will need 5–7g/kg BW during this 24-hour period. As a rule of thumb, stick to a fist-size portion of a complex carbohydrate choice 4–6 times during the day. In food terms this will look like:

>>> 50g (1³⁄₄oz) rolled oats

>>> Banana

>>> Fist-size portion of sweet potato

>>> 3–4 oatcakes

>>> Fist-size portion of cooked rice/couscous

>>> Piece of toast

This little and often approach is important as it allows for more efficient glycogen storage and causes less stomach discomfort or problems during your long ride. Getting into the habit of this fuelling strategy will be beneficial for competition day too. Have a look at the endurance training sample menus in Chapter 2 to become more familiar with this type of fuelling. Once you've sorted your pre-training nutrition, it is time to think about what you might need during your ride.

Remember, these rides are not high intensity so they don't need carbohydrate as an available fuel source. By using the fuelling strategy described earlier in this section, you will have full glycogen stores. These full stores will provide you with fuel for around 90 minutes to 2 hours at a low–moderate intensity pace. Once this has been used up, your body will switch to fat stores within the body to enable you to continue cycling. As carbohydrate is not a necessary fuel in these situations, I always advise people to choose food/snacks that they will want to eat en route. When you are out cycling for this length of time, it becomes a mental challenge as well as a physical one and if you have little treats/snacks that you are looking forward to eating, you are more likely to complete your cycle successfully.

> **Tip** *During endurance rides over 3 hours you will need 60g of carbohydrate per hour. Try alternating between fast-release choices such as energy gels, jelly babies and dried fruit with slower-release real-food options, such as yeast extract sandwiches, Banana and Nut Butter Sandwich (see page 267); Sweet Potato Brownies (see page 264) or salted peanuts every 45 minutes.*

DON'T FORGET TO HYDRATE

If it is hot, take electrolytes (see page 37) or add a quarter teaspoon of table salt to every 500ml/17fl oz of squash. This will help to replace salt losses through sweat, while helping you to draw more water into your body and stay hydrated. If you choose to use energy drinks or squash with added sugar, remember that they are providing you with carbohydrate and you will need to adjust your food intake accordingly. Your body can only absorb a maximum of 90g/3oz of carbohydrate an hour so over-consuming carbohydrate can cause stomach discomfort/ problems in some individuals.

HIGH-INTENSITY TRAINING

These training sessions are going to be done very close to or above your lactate threshold (see page 55). Remember the key to these sessions is to improve your lactate threshold, meaning that you will be able to ride at a faster speed for longer before it becomes too difficult to maintain due to acid build-up.

Some examples of high-intensity training sessions include:

>>> Hill sessions such as 5 x 8: this involves riding up a hill for 5 minutes, recovering by descending to the bottom and repeating 8 times, with a 10-minute warm up and cool-down ride at an easy pace. This session is building on strength and endurance and is going to feel hard; you will not be able to have a conversation while riding up the hill.

>>> Flat interval 5 x 5; this will be riding flat out so at around 80–90 percent of your maximal heart rate for 5 minutes with a 90-second recovery, repeated 5 times, with a 10-minute warm up and cool-down ride at easy pace. This session could also been done as a turbo or spinning bike session.

>>> 60-minute threshold ride: warm up with a 10-minute easy-pace ride and then increase your pace to 75 percent of your maximal heart rate, which will be around your lactate threshold. Maintain this pace for 40 minutes. At this threshold pace you should be able to talk but

may struggle to get more than five words out, with three words being manageable. Cool down with a 10-minute easy-pace ride. Again this session can be done on a turbo or spin bike.

FUEL REQUIREMENTS

These high-intensity training sessions need carbohydrate. You will be unable to do this type of session without it in your system. Your daily requirements of carbohydrate will be as high as 5g/kg BW in females and 7g/kg BW in males. This equates to 5–7 fist-size portions of carbohydrate distributed throughout the day as meals and snacks. You will also need 4–6 palm-size portions or 0.25g/kg BW protein.

If you are planning to do this training session in the morning, pay attention to consuming carbohydrate in your main meal the night before. Aim for 1–2g/kg BW as a serving size. Follow this up with a similar portion at breakfast at least 1–2 hours before you plan to train.

If you are planning to do this type of session in the evening, ensure you consume 1g/kg BW carbohydrate at breakfast, lunch and a pre-training snack prior to the session.

Have a look at the high-intensity sample menus in Chapter 2 to see how you can ensure you meet your fuelling needs, depending on when you are training.

After such a hard session, recovery is going to be important. If you have a session within 12 hours, then ensure recovery is within 30 minutes of finishing the session and includes 1.2g/kg BW carbohydrate and 0.25g/kg BW protein in a liquid form with fast-acting carbohydrate and easily digestible protein. A good option is flavoured milk or a Mocha Shake (see page 277).

If your next training session is over 12 hours, ensure recovery is within 2 hours of finishing this session and includes 1.2g/kg BW carbohydrate and 0.25g/kg BW protein as a meal. Try Half and Half Chilli Con Carne (see page 232).

PLANNING YOUR TRAINING WEEK

Although it is important to fuel each training day according to the type of session, you also need to think about how this all flows together in a week. In the sample week overleaf, Tuesday, Wednesday and Saturday are low-intensity or rest days, so your body doesn't require carbohydrate for energy. However, each one is before a high-intensity or endurance ride, which means that sufficient carbohydrate is needed in preparation. The easiest way to do this is to have a carbohydrate-based meal on Tuesday and Wednesday evening. Similarly, you should aim to eat small regular amounts of carbohydrate throughout Saturday, ready for Sunday. You will also need to pay special attention to your recovery by having carbohydrate and protein meals or snacks every 2–3 hours on Sunday in preparation for Monday's high-intensity session.

Day of the week	Training intensity
Monday	60 mins high intensity
Tuesday	60 mins low-intensity recovery ride building on aerobic base
Wednesday	Rest
Thursday	80 mins high intensity
Friday	90 mins moderate-intensity bike ride keeping a constant pace
Saturday	Rest
Sunday	3-hour-plus low-moderate intensity endurance ride

TABLE 3.4 A sample training week

CASE STUDY

My client was a man who initially contacted me because he was commuting 56km/35 miles to work by bike and did not feel he was meeting his requirements appropriately. Ideally he wanted to commute daily but was only managing three days a week. He was too fatigued by Wednesday evening to continue cycling that week. He was also constantly hungry but struggling to shift a few stubborn pounds, despite cycling over 160km/100 miles a week.

His typical day's food intake was as follows:

Pre-morning bike ride: Bowl of Coco Pops
At work after shower, at desk: Bacon sandwich, packet of crisps

Lunch:	2 chicken mayonnaise and salad wraps; large chocolate bar
Pre-afternoon bike ride:	Cereal bar and handful jelly babies
Home:	Large portion of pasta with sauce, cheese and garlic bread; bowl of ice cream; crackers and cheese

The main issue was that he was consuming what I call a 'reactive diet'. He was making poor choices, high in quick-release carbohydrate, which were causing blood-sugar fluctuations, making him reach for more high-sugar foods and leaving him fatigued.

The first thing we discussed was recovery. I explained that by making a good recovery choice after his morning commute, he would immediately start the glycogen re-building process. This would ensure he would have enough fuel for his afternoon commute home. I also advised that he included more complex carbohydrate and lean protein choices in his daily intake, which would help to keep his blood-sugar and energy levels more stable, as well as providing him with important nutrients to meet his training/commuting needs.

His revised example daily plan looked as follows:

Pre-morning bike ride:	Smoothie
At work after shower, at desk:	300–500ml/10½–17fl oz chocolate milk, followed by wholegrain bagel with peanut butter and banana or similar
Lunch:	Jacket potato with tuna and salad, yogurt
Mid-afternoon:	2 hot-cross buns and 75g/2½oz mixed nuts
Post-afternoon bike ride:	500ml/17fl oz milk
6.30pm:	Main meal followed by natural yogurt with fruit and honey
9.30pm:	Hot chocolate with oatcakes and peanut butter

Initially he was not convinced that this change in style of eating was actually going to make a big difference to his 'insatiable hunger', as he had described it. However, a few weeks later

> I received an email from him reporting that all was more than well on the new plan. He was feeling much better at work, able to concentrate and had more energy.
>
> He was now riding his bike four times a week and was working up to doing it five times. He had lost those few stubborn pounds and he had also signed up to do his first 100-mile sportive in 3 months time.

SWIMMING

Swimmers routinely train for long and usually anti-social hours; elite swimmers can be training for as much as 6 hours a day in a heavy training block, including a mix of pool and land training in the form of strength and conditioning.

Training will be 4–10 sessions a week, covering varying distances. Sprinters typically have lower training volumes, covering less distance but often at much higher speeds and intensities than distance or open-water swimmers, who can travel up to 10K per session at lower speeds.

STARTING YOUNG

Due to the nature of swimming, it is not uncommon to start training at a young age, with training commitments being high in late adolescence into the teens. Juggling early morning training with school, while also trying to meet growth and training demands, has huge nutritional implications. See The Young Athlete in Chapter 1, page 28.

Weekly training plans for swimmers will include sessions at different intensities. As with all sports, nutritional intake has to match the demands of these different training intensity sessions.

In Chapter 2 we looked at RPE (Rate of Perceived Exertion) to help you train at the right intensities and fuel these sessions appropriately. In swimming this use of RPE is even more important, as heart rates tend to be up to 13 beats lower in the water – this means working to heart rate might not be as useful as it is in other sports. Table 3.5 below recaps RPE scale swimming. Table 3.6 shows a typical swimming training week.

Intensity	How this feels	RPE
Easy	Relaxed, easy	5/10
Moderate	Comfortable, controlled	6–7/10
High	Challenging and becoming harder as the session progresses	8–9/10

TABLE 3.5 The RPE (rate of perceived exertion) scale

Day of the week	Training intensity
Monday	30 mins easy-intensity recovery swim
Tuesday	60 mins moderate-intensity drills
Wednesday	Rest or strength training
Thursday	60 mins high-intensity intervals
Friday	45 mins moderate-intensity, keeping a constant speed
Saturday	Rest or strength training
Sunday	2-hour swim session with easy-moderate drills

TABLE 3.6 A typical training week

So let's look at some examples of actual training sessions and their nutritional demands.

LOW-INTENSITY TRAINING

Regardless of what distance you are training for, a low-intensity recovery swim will always be the same format. It will be a maximum of 60 minutes swimming at an easy pace, working at a RPE of 5/10 in any stroke. It is the pace where you swim easily and if it was possible practically, you could have a conversation at the same time! You will feel more energized after this type of swim, making it useful to put in between two harder sessions.

FUEL REQUIREMENTS

A low-intensity easy swim has no fuel demands as long as the session is kept to a maximum of 60 minutes. A great time to do these easy swims is first thing in the morning in a fasted state, as your body will obtain what it needs from your fat or glycogen stores. That said, these easy-pace swims can be done at any time that works for you but there is no need for any specific fuelling strategy in preparation.

So on a day when you are doing an easy-pace, low-intensity swim, your maximum carbohydrate requirements are 3g/kg BW and your protein requirements will be 3–4 servings of 0.25g/kg BW a day. This can be easily achieved by sticking to three meals a day, combining fist-size portions of complex carbohydrate foods, such as oats, sweet potato, root vegetables or pulses, with a palm-size portion of protein such as eggs, chicken or fish, served with unlimited undressed salad or vegetables. Snack on fruit or vegetables.

Hydration is also really important for swimmers. Swimming pools are often warm, humid environments. Moderate sweat losses might not be obvious to you as you are already wet. Keep a bottle of water at the poolside and take sips regularly. In very hot conditions, aim for 200ml/7fl oz every 20 minutes.

Take some time to refer back to the low-intensity sample menus in Chapter 2. These are really helpful in demonstrating how to meet the nutritional requirements for low-intensity training and rest days. They incorporate recipes from this book, which are suitable to serve up to the whole family while still making sure you're meeting your training needs.

· ·

ARE SWIMMERS THE HUNGRIEST ATHLETES?

A national nutritional survey of athletes from a range of sports a few years ago reported that swimmers tended to have higher appetites and energy intakes than other athletes. Indeed, I see this frequently in practice too. In order to explain this, many studies have been conducted and, although there doesn't seem to be an absolutely conclusive answer, the most likely explanation is that swimming doesn't cause the appetite drop that accompanies heavy running and cycling training. Many of you may have observed that feeling of 'eating like a horse' after you have finished a swim training session. Some research suggests that this is due to the cool temperatures in which swimmers train. By contrast, runners and cyclists usually experience an increase in body temperature during training, which may serve to suppress appetite – at least in the short term. Due to this, care needs to be taken, especially in these low-intensity training sessions that you do not over-compensate for the energy you have just burned.

One good tip that I have found works with a lot of swimmers is to encourage them to have a hot drink as soon as possible after they have left the pool. This helps to bring core temperature back up and helps them make more suitable nutritional choices post-training.

●●●

MODERATE-INTENSITY TRAINING

When doing moderate-intensity training, you will feel like you are holding a comfortable pace, working at 6–7/10 on the RPE scale.

Some scenarios include:

>>> 45–60-minute constant swim at this moderate intensity in the stroke that you are competing in. Halfway through the session think about your 'kick'; aim to kick for 100m as hard as you can and have a goal time to aim for. This way you can check your progression weekly. Always remember to warm up and cool down with a 100m easy pace in any stroke.

>>> Moderate-intensity swim session with drills. Warm up with 100m easy pace in any stroke, followed by 30 seconds rest and then 8 sets of 4 x 25m at a moderate intensity with 10 seconds rest between each 25m and a 3-minute rest between each set in a competing stroke. Cool down with a 100m easy swim in any stroke.

FUEL REQUIREMENTS
This session is harder than an easy swim but it is still within your comfort zone. Your daily carbohydrate requirement will be

a maximum of 5g/kg BW and your protein requirement will be 0.25g/kg BW four times a day. The moderate-intensity sample menu plans in Chapter 2 demonstrate what these requirements look like and also take into account the time of day you swim.

If you are an experienced swimmer, you may feel confident to do this moderate-intensity session early morning in a fasted state but ensure you are hydrated and keep the session to a maximum of 60 minutes.

If, however, this session is going to be over 60 minutes, or is scheduled for the day after a hard training session, you will need to have some fuel before your swim. Some good examples include:

>>> Banana

>>> 1–2 pieces of malt loaf

>>> 1 piece of toast

>>> Small pot of fat-free Greek yogurt with 1–2 tsp honey

Take time to think about your recovery needs after your swim. Aim for 1g/kg BW carbohydrate and 0.25g/kg BW protein and also bear in mind the time frame.

If this is your only training session for the day, aim to eat this recovery meal or snack within 2 hours of completing your swim. For most of you this will fall at your next meal.

For example, you go out for a moderate-intensity training session before breakfast at 6.30am and return at 7.30am. You are not planning on doing any further training today. The key is to have a good recovery breakfast, such as Scrambled Egg Pitta (see page 192) or Sunflower Seed and Chia Porridge (see page 188) by 9.30am. Both of these suggestions are hot breakfasts, which will help to get your core temperature back up to normal. It's your choice if you want to have this as you walk back through the door or if you would prefer to have a shower first!

If you are planning to do a second training session within the next 12 hours and your next meal is not imminent after this run, you will need a recovery choice such as the Recovery Hot Chocolate (see page 277) within 30 minutes, followed by a meal 2 hours later.

ENDURANCE TRAINING

The endurance swim is a 2-hour session at an easy pace, with moderate drills to help break up the session and encourage you to develop your kick and stroke technique.

So within your 2-hour easy swim you will include moderate-intensity drills, such as:

>>> 8 x 50m at RPE 6–7/10 of competing stroke with 15 seconds rest after each 50m

>>> 400m swim continuous swimming at RPE 6–7/10 in competing stroke with an explosive sprint finish in the last 15m; continue with an easy pace swim in a competing stroke

Nutritionally these endurance swims are demanding and glycogen stores will be depleted. You will need to prepare 24 hours prior to these swims, taking on sufficient amounts of carbohydrate, as well as during.

FUEL REQUIREMENTS

The key nutrition strategy for endurance training is to consume small amounts of carbohydrate in the 24 hours before every meal and snack. You will need 5–7g/kg BW during this 24-hour period. As a rule of thumb, stick to a fist-size portion of a complex carbohydrate 4–6 times during the day. Visually this will look like:

>>> 50g/1¾oz rolled oats

>>> Banana

>>> Fist-size piece of sweet potato

>>> 3–4 oatcakes

>>> Fist-size portion of cooked rice/couscous

>>> Piece of toast

This little and often approach is important as it allows for more efficient glycogen storage and causes less stomach discomfort or problems during your long swim. Getting into the habit of this fuelling strategy will be beneficial for competition day too. Even if your chosen distance is 100m, swimming competitions tend to have several heats. It is important to fuel correctly to ensure that you have sufficient energy for all your heats. Look at the endurance training sample menus in Chapter 2 to become more familiar with this type of fuelling.

Once you've sorted out your pre-training nutrition, it is time to think about what you might need during your swim. This can be complicated as many swimmers prefer not to stop to eat anything. The simplest and most practical way to get round this is to keep an energy drink at the poolside and take regular sips.

If you have followed the nutrition strategy and met your needs in the 24 hours prior to these 2-hour endurance swims, you will have full glycogen stores. These full stores will be sufficient to provide energy for 90 minutes to 2 hours at low-moderate intensity.

> **Tip**
> 500ml/17fl oz of any sports drink, branded or the homemade version in Chapter 2 (see page 80), will provide you with 500ml/17fl oz of fluid, 140 calories, 30g of carbohydrate and 250mg of sodium, which is ideal to keep stores topped up during this training session.

HIGH-INTENSITY TRAINING

High-intensity training sessions are going to be done very close to or above your lactate threshold. Remember the key is to improve your lactate threshold, meaning that you will be able to swim at a faster speed for your required distance before it becomes too difficult to maintain due to acid build-up. In swimming, because many distances such as 50m freestyle or 200m breaststroke will be completed within 3 minutes, these high-intensity sessions are also going to help to build your anaerobic metabolism, particularly glycolysis (see page 54). These sessions will be challenging and feel hard. Some examples of high-intensity training scenarios include:

>>> 200m warm-up at an easy pace in any stroke, rest for 30 seconds;
4 x 25m working at 8–9/10 RPE with 30 seconds rest between each 25m
in competition stroke; followed by an easy pace for 200m; 8 x 25m
working at 8–9/10 RPE with 15 seconds recovery between each 25m in
competition stroke. Repeat this whole sequence three times.

>>> Warm up with an easy pace of any stroke for 500m; followed by
500m continuous hard swimming in competition stroke working
8–9/10 RPE; 200m easy pace in competition stroke; 400m continuous
hard swimming in competition stroke; 200m recovery in easy stroke;
300m continuous hard; 200m recovery easy pace; 200m hard; 200m
recovery; 100m hard; 3 minutes recovery. Finish with 8 x 25m hard with
15 seconds recovery between each 25m. Cool down with 300m
easy pace.

FUEL REQUIREMENTS

You will be unable to do this type of high-intensity session without
carbohydrate in your system. Your daily requirement of carbohydrate
will be as high as 5g/kg BW in females and 7g/kg BW in males.
This equates to 5–7 fist-size portions of carbohydrate distributed
throughout the day as meals and snacks. You will also need 4–6 palm-
size portions or 0.25g/kg BW protein.

If you are planning to do this session in the morning, pay
attention to consuming carbohydrate in your main meal the night
before, aiming for 1–2g/kg BW as a serving size. Follow this up with
a similar portion at breakfast at least 1–2 hours before you plan
on training.

If you are planning to do this type of session in the evening,
ensure you have 1g/kg BW carbohydrate at breakfast, lunch and a
pre-training snack prior to the session.

Look at the high-intensity sample menus in Chapter 2 to see how
you can ensure you meet your fuel needs, depending on when you
are training.

After such a hard session, recovery is going to be important.
As previously highlighted in Chapter 2, if you have a session within
12 hours, ensure recovery is within 30 minutes of finishing this
session and includes 1.2g/kg BW carbohydrate and 0.25g/kg BW
protein in a liquid form, with fast-acting carbohydrate and easily
digestible protein. A good choice is Recovery Hot Chocolate (see
page 277), which has the added benefit of helping to bring the core
temperature back up to normal.

If your next training session is over 12 hours, ensure recovery is within 2 hours of finishing this session and includes 1.2g/kg BW carbohydrate and 0.25g/kg BW protein as a meal. A good choice is Chicken and Cannellini Stroganoff (see page 226).

•••

OPEN-WATER SWIMMING

The popularity of open-water swimming has risen since 2008, when it was included as an Olympic sport at the Beijing games.

Open-water races can take place in any large outdoor body of water: seas, lakes, rivers, canals and reservoirs. The distance of each event varies from 1km to 80km, but at the major competitive level, the typical distances are 5km, 10km and 25km. Elite swimmers will complete a 5K event close to the hour mark and a 10K in around 2 hours. So for those of you who are serious recreational open-water swimmers, it will take slightly longer in both distances.

There are numerous other factors to consider with open-water swimming; firstly, you are most likely to compete wearing a wetsuit, which is going to affect your buoyancy in the water and your swim technique. Secondly, very cold water can cause breathing difficulties in even the most experience swimmers and, finally, rough conditions will add resistance, using up total energy stores, and in some individuals can also cause 'sea sickness', which will need to be overcome.

As in all sports, matching your nutritional intake to your training and competition needs is going to have real benefits to your overall performance. So think about your next training session:

>>> How long is it going to be?

>>> How intense is it going to be?

Then you can start preparing for it. Let's take a 10K open-water swim as an example. This is going to last over 90 minutes and so the nutritional strategies you would put in place for endurance swims (see page 133) are going to apply. Make sure you fuel adequately in the 24 hours prior to this session so that you have full glycogen stores. Fuelling during a 10K training session could be more complicated. As with the endurance swim, combining energy needs with hydration is going to be the ideal solution. However, this will only be possible if you are training in an open-water body where you either have boat support to offer you a drink or are within a lake/reservoir where there is a landing stage for drinks.

During a 10k competition, it is advisable to aim for 30–60g carbohydrate an hour, aiming to start taking on your nutrition in the first 45 minutes to delay the onset of fatigue by sparing your glycogen stores.

Some good strategies include:

>>> Fuelling every lap – 8 x 1,250m lap (eight opportunities to feed). Over eight feed stations, to consume 60g carbohydrate you would need to have 15g at every station, which is 300ml/10½fl oz of a standard sports drink.

>>> If you do not want to fuel at every station, try boosting the carbohydrate content of your drink. You can do this by mixing in a gel or additional sports drink powder to get the desired carbohydrate content but remember to taste-test and practise in training to avoid any stomach discomfort.

Once the race is over, recovery nutrition should be consumed as soon as is possible, and definitely within 2 hours of finishing. Aim for 1g/kg BW carbohydrate and 0.25g/kg BW protein. 500ml/17fl oz of flavoured milk is ideal as it also helps replace fluid and electrolytes. Alternatively a chicken sandwich and a fruit smoothie would also work well (see page 87 for Endurance Training meal planner ideas).

Keep hydrating with small frequent drinks, and if it is a particularly hot day try to consume small amounts of foods that are high in salt such as cheese, salted peanuts or yeast extract on toast.

PLANNING YOUR TRAINING WEEK

Although it is important to fuel each training day according to the type of session, you also need to think about how this all flows together in a week. In the example overleaf, Monday, Wednesday and Saturday are low-intensity or rest days, so your body doesn't require carbohydrate for energy. However, each one is before a day when you will be doing a moderate-intensity, high-intensity or endurance session, which means you need to consume sufficient carbohydrate in preparation. The easiest way to do this is to have a carbohydrate-based meal on Monday and Wednesday evening. Similarly, you should aim to eat small, regular amounts of carbohydrate throughout Saturday, ready for Sunday.

Day of the week	Training intensity
Monday	30 mins easy-intensity recovery swim
Tuesday	60 mins moderate-intensity drills
Wednesday	Rest or strength training
Thursday	60 mins high-intensity intervals
Friday	45 mins moderate intensity, keeping a constant speed
Saturday	Rest or strength training
Sunday	2-hour swim session with easy-moderate drills

TABLE 3.7 A typical training week

CASE STUDY

My client was a 15-year-old female swimmer, who had started swimming at nine years old and had been swimming competitively since she was 12. Her distance and stroke was 50m/100m backstroke.

Her goal was to achieve a personal best (PB) of under 1.06 minutes in 100m to qualify for the nationals. She knew that to do this she had to reduce her body fat composition, as this would help her to sit better in the water and prevent drag. She also reported that she was struggling with light-headedness and trembling around training.

She was training six days a week. On four of these days she trained twice a day with each session being 1–2 hours. Additionally she was juggling her training around attending school and doing coursework. Her nutritional issues were:

>>> Poor planning – she made unsuitable nutritional choices before her early morning training sessions and recovery, before rushing off to school.

>>> Her packed lunch was full of high-fat, high-sugar, fast-release carbohydrate foods such as crisps, cereal bars, and white pitta bread with cheese.

>>> Although she ate a main meal before her evening training session, she was often very hungry and snacked on toast with chocolate spread and biscuits before going to bed.

It was the constant fuelling with high-sugar foods that was causing her to feel tired and shaky during training sessions. In addition, her poor recovery choices meant that her glycogen stores were not replenished sufficiently before her evening training session.

My advice was as follows:

>>> To concentrate on good recovery snacks – this was particularly important because she had 12 hours or less between training sessions. Making the right meal choices to support her training would prevent fatigue, improve performance and provide body composition gains.

>>> Carbohydrate requirement – 3–5g/kg BW but it needed be altered according to her training schedule.

>>> Protein requirement – 0.25g/kg BW, aiming for some protein foods with every meal to help maintain stable sugar levels; this was also extremely important post-training.

>>> Before training, aim for carbohydrate-rich snacks or meals, 1–3 hours before, depending on tolerance.

>>> After training, especially if the next session is less than 8 hours, recovery needs to start as quickly as possible, 15–30 minutes after the session has finished. This should be a mix of carbohydrate and protein.

I suggested the following sample menu:

Pre-training:	Fruit smoothie or a fruit yogurt and banana
During swim:	Homemade sports drink – 250ml/9fl oz orange juice, 250ml/9fl oz water with ¼ tsp salt
Post-training:	1 piece wholemeal or rye toast with 2 scrambled eggs and 250ml/9fl oz skimmed milk
11am:	Fruit
Lunch:	Chicken salad with couscous; yogurt
Pre-training:	2 crumpets with honey, or a bowl of cereal, or 2 pieces malt loaf
Post-training:	500ml/17fl oz chocolate milk in the car on the way home
6.30pm:	Sausage Casserole (see page 235)
Post-training:	500ml/17fl oz chocolate milk in the car on the way home
9.30pm:	Fruit and yogurt

She came for a follow-up appointment six weeks later. Her weight had dropped by 3kg/6lb and her body fat percentage by 2 percent. She had seen huge improvements in her performance and was getting closer to her PB. She no longer struggled with trembling, dizziness or fatigue.

COMBINE AND CONQUER: TRIATHLON

Triathlon is a sport involving three disciplines: swimming, cycling and running, as a continuous race over various distances. See Table 3.8 (opposite) for examples of the different types of triathlon. There is a transition period between the disciplines, which is an integral part of the race.

Type	Swim length	Cycle length	Run length
Super sprint	400m	10K	2.5K
Sprint	750m	20K	5K
Standard	1500m	40K	10K
Middle	2.5K	80K	20K
Ironman	3.8K	180K	42K

TABLE 3.8 Types of triathlon

Triathlons, regardless of distance, are endurance activities, where you need to have the physique and physiological make-up suited to all three disciplines. This can be challenging. Finding time to train across all three sports and preventing fatigue contributed by both the physical and psychological demands of this multi-sport event makes appropriate training and nutritional strategies fundamental to success.

Meeting your training needs nutritionally will have positive implications on overall performance. Training will involve sessions working just above and below your lactate threshold in all three disciplines, as well as low-intensity recovery sessions and endurance sessions of the individual sports as well as combinations. One such example is a BRICK session, which includes a cycling session followed immediately by a run, which helps the body to adapt to using different muscle groups.

	Monday	Tuesday	Wednesday	Thursday	Friday	Saturday	Sunday
Swim	45 mins moderate-intensity intervals before work	60 mins low intensity before work	Rest	45 mins high-intensity intervals before work	1.5K swim technique	Rest	45 mins low-intensity recovery swim in the evening
Bike	Spin class at lunchtime (45 mins high intensity)	Rest	Spin class at lunchtime (45 mins high intensity)	Rest	Rest	BRICK session – Long bike ride (60 mins low to moderate intensity)	Long bike ride in morning with club 50k
Run	Rest	Track session with club pm – high-intensity intervals (60 mins)	Hilly run with club pm (60 mins moderate intensity)	45 mins low-intensity recovery run after work	Rest	Followed by 60 mins run low to moderate intensity total time 2 hours	Rest

TABLE 3.2 A weekly training schedule for a triathlon

Don't worry too much about which of the three disciplines you are doing; focus on the intensity and length of that training and ensure that you fuel up correctly around that session. The information in the rest of this section will enable you to do this correctly. Let's look at some examples of actual training sessions and their nutritional demands.

> **Tip**
> *As you are likely to have less than 12 hours recovery between training sessions (morning and then evening, or evening then morning), you will need to pay specific attention to your recovery choices to ensure that your body has sufficient energy for the second session of the day.*

LOW-INTENSITY TRAINING

Regardless of which of the three disciplines you are training for – swimming, cycling or running – a low-intensity training session will always be the same format. It will be a maximum of 60 minutes at an easy pace. It is the pace at which you are still able to have a conversation while you train! You will feel more energized after this type of session, making it useful to put in between two harder sessions.

Some examples in all three disciplines include:

>>> Maximum 60-minute swim, any stroke working at an RPE of 5/10

>>> Maximum of 60 minutes ride at an easy pace – around 50 percent of your maximal heart rate and building on your overall aerobic endurance

>>> Maximum of 60 minutes run at an easy pace – around 50 percent of your maximal heart rate. The run will be between 90 seconds to 2 minutes slower than your race pace; it should always be slower, never quicker

FUEL REQUIREMENTS

A low-intensity training session has no fuel demands. A great time to do these sessions is first thing in the morning in a fasted state, as your body will obtain what it needs from your fat or glycogen stores. That said, these easy-pace sessions can be done at any time that works for you but, whenever you do them, there is no need for any specific fuelling strategy in preparation.

So on a day when you are *only* doing an easy pace, low-intensity training session and are not following up with a second session later in the day, your maximum carbohydrate requirement will be 3g/kg BW and your protein requirement will be 3–4 servings of 0.25g/kg BW a day. This can be easily achieved by sticking to three meals a day, combining fist-size portions of complex carbohydrate foods, such as oats, sweet potato, root vegetables or pulses, with a palm-size portion of protein, such as eggs, chicken or fish, served with unlimited undressed salad or vegetables. Snack on fruit or vegetables.

It is, however, most likely when training for a triathlon that you will do a further session later in the day. In these cases, your carbohydrate requirement is actually going to be 5–7g/kg BW, so 4–6 fist-size servings and 4–6 servings of 0.25g/kg BW protein.

You will also need to consume your recovery nutrition within 30 minutes of finishing your first training session to start the replenishing process, ensuring that you have sufficient energy for your second session of the day.

> **Tip** *It is very important to maintain hydration throughout the day. Drink little and often and ensure that your urine is pale straw in colour.*

Take some time to refer back to the low-intensity sample menus in Chapter 2. These are really helpful in demonstrating how to meet the nutritional requirements for a low-intensity training day. They incorporate recipes from this book, which are suitable to serve up to the whole family while still making sure your are meeting your training needs.

If, however, you are doing two training sessions in one day, the following plans are more relevant:

Sample Menu plan 1

60 MINS LOW-INTENSITY SESSION

Breakfast: Scrambled Egg Pitta (see page 192) (eat within 30 minutes of completing session)

Snack: Banana

45 MINS HIGH-INTENSITY SESSION

Lunch: Sweet Potato and Red Lentil Soup (see page 212); slice of Lemon Drizzle Polenta Cake (see page 289)

Snack: Cranberry and Mango Smoothie (see page 183)

Dinner: Easy Fish and Chips (see page 247); Mango and Kiwi Baskets (see page 284); Recovery Hot Chocolate (see page 277)

Sample Menu Plan 2

Breakfast: Buckwheat Pancakes with Strawberries and Vanilla
                   Yogurt (see page 194)
45 MINS HIGH-INTENSITY SESSION
Post-training: 250ml/9fl oz flavoured milk
Lunch: Hearty Vegetable Soup (see page 210) with Cheese and
                   Chilli Scone (see page 273)
Snack: Banana
40 MINS MODERATE-INTENSITY SESSION
Dinner: Magic Fish Pie (see page 248); Rhubarb Granola
                   Crumble (see page 290)

Sample Menu Plan 3

30 MINS MODERATE-INTENSITY SESSION
Breakfast: Scrambled Egg Pitta (see page 192)
Lunch: Three-Lentil Dhal with Coriander and Chilli
                   (see page 213)
Snack: Dark Chocolate and Ginger Muffin (see page 260)
30 MINS MODERATE-INTENSITY SESSION
Dinner: Sweet Potato Parcels (see page 254); Summer Fruit and
                   Mint Kebabs (see page 283) or a fruit salad

MODERATE-INTENSITY TRAINING

These moderate-intensity training sessions will look a little different
depending on which of the triathlon disciplines you are doing. Some
training scenarios might include:

>>> **Run:** A moderate-intensity training session will be a 'tempo' run.
    These sessions take the format of a 10-minute warm up, immediately
    followed by 20–40 minutes at a faster pace, about 30 seconds
    slower than your race pace and close to your lactate threshold. This
    tempo pace will feel hard but controlled; you won't be able to talk
    comfortably but it should not feel as if you're racing.

>>> **Bike:** Moderate-intensity training rides usually take the format of a
    'steady state', varying in time from 60–90 minutes. This is faster than
    your 'easy' pace. You should be able to carry on a conversation but

may have to occasionally take an extra breath between sentences. If you use a heart-rate monitor, it will be working at around 60–70 percent of your maximal heart rate. These sessions can be done on the road, or on a turbo trainer or spinning bike but remember to keep to the right intensity.

>>> **Bike:** A moderate-intensity swim session with drills. Warm up with 100m easy pace in any stroke; 30 seconds rest and then 8 sets of 4 x 25m at a moderate intensity, RPE 6–7/10 with 10 seconds rest between each 25m and 3 minutes rest between each set in a competing stroke. Cool down with 100m easy swim in any stroke.

FUEL REQUIREMENTS

These sessions are harder than an easy session but you will still be training within your comfort zone. Your daily carbohydrate requirements will be a maximum of 5g/kg BW and your protein requirement will be 0.25g/kg BW four times a day. The moderate-intensity sample menu plans in Chapter 2 demonstrate what this look likes practically and also take into account the time of day you do your training.

If you have trained regularly for a while, you may feel confident enough to do these moderate-intensity sessions early morning in a fasted state but do ensure you are hydrated and keep the session to a maximum of 60 minutes.

If, however, this session is going to be 60–90 minutes or is scheduled after a hard training session, you will need to have some fuel before. Some good examples include:

>>> Banana

>>> 1–2 pieces of malt loaf

>>> 1 piece of toast

>>> Small pot of fat-free Greek yogurt with 1–2 tsp honey

After your run, take time to think about your recovery needs. Aim for 1g/kg BW carbohydrate and 0.25g/kg BW protein and also the time frame. If this is your only training session for the day, aim to eat this recovery meal or snack within 2 hours of completing your run. This may fall at your next meal.

For example, you go out for a steady state run before breakfast at 6.30am and return at 7.30am. You are not planning on doing any further training today. The key is to have a good recovery breakfast, such as Blueberry Bircher Muesli (see page 185) or Scrambled Egg Pitta (see page 192) by 9.30am. It's your choice if you want to have this as you walk back through the door or if you would prefer to have a shower first!

If you are planning on a second training session within the next 12 hours and your next meal is not imminent after this run, you will need a recovery choice such as the Tropical Smoothie (see page 276) within 30 minutes followed by a meal 2 hours later.

ENDURANCE TRAINING

These are all your sessions over 90 minutes, whether this is a BRICK session (cycling then running) or individual sports, most likely if you are training for an Ironman event. Three example scenarios are:

1. **2-hour bike ride at an easy to moderate pace followed immediately by a 1-hour easy pace run**

2. **50K long ride over a hilly route**

3. **5–10K open-water swim at an easy pace**

Nutritionally these endurance sessions are demanding, as glycogen stores will be depleted. You will need to prepare 24 hours prior to these sessions, taking on sufficient amounts of carbohydrate, as well as during.

FUEL REQUIREMENTS

The key nutrition strategy for endurance training is to consume small amounts of carbohydrate in the 24 hours before every meal and snack. As a rule of thumb, stick to a fist-size portion of a complex carbohydrate 4–6 times during the day. Visually this will look like:

>>> 50g/1¾ oz rolled oats

>>> Banana

>>> Fist-size portion of sweet potato

>>> 3–4 oatcakes

>>> Fist-size portion of cooked rice/couscous

>>> Piece of toast

This little and often approach is important as it allows for more efficient glycogen storage and causes less stomach discomfort or problems during your endurance session. Getting into the habit of this fuelling strategy will be beneficial for race day too. Look at the endurance training sample menus in Chapter 2 to become more familiar with this type of fuelling. Once you've sorted your pre-training nutrition, it is time to think about what you might need during your ride.

Remember these sessions are not high intensity, so they don't need carbohydrate as an available fuel source; by using the fuelling strategy above, you will have full glycogen stores. These full stores will provide you with fuel for around 90 minutes to 2 hours at a low-moderate intensity pace. Once this has been used up, your body will switch to fat stores to enable you to keep training. As carbohydrate is not a necessary fuel in these situations, I advise people to choose foods that they will want to eat en route. When you are out training for this length of time, it becomes a mental challenge as well as a physical one. If you have little treats and snacks that you are looking forward to, you are more likely to complete your training successfully.

(Tip)

During endurance sessions over 3 hours you will need 60g of carbohydrate an hour. Try alternating between fast-release carbohydrate choices such as energy gels, jelly babies and dried fruit and slower-release real-food options such as yeast extract sandwiches, Banana and Nut Butter Sandwich (see page 267), Sweet Potato Brownies (see page 264) or salted peanuts every 45 minutes.

Don't forget to hydrate. If it is hot, take electrolytes or add a quarter teaspoon of table salt to every 500ml/17fl oz of squash. This will help replace salt losses through sweat while helping you to draw more water into your body and stay hydrated. If you choose to use energy drinks or squash with added sugar, remember that they are providing you with carbohydrate and you will need to adjust your food intake accordingly. Your body can only absorb a maximum of 90g/3oz of carbohydrate an hour, so over-consuming hourly carbohydrate can cause stomach discomfort/problems in some individuals.

HIGH-INTENSITY TRAINING

These training sessions will be done very close to or above your lactate threshold. Remember, the key to these sessions is to improve your lactate threshold, meaning that you will be able to run/swim/bike at a faster speed for longer before it becomes too difficult to maintain due to acid build-up. Here are three training scenarios, based on the different disciplines:

>>> **Run:** 6 x 6 minutes with 2 minutes recovery between each 6-minute effort. As each effort is 6 minutes you will be challenging your lactate threshold, breathing hard but controlled so that you can keep this pace for the 6 minutes. If you start these efforts too hard, you will struggle to keep a constant pace over the six efforts. By repeating this session week after week, the aim will be that eventually these 6-minute efforts will be run at a faster pace, meaning that you have increased your lactate threshold.

>>> **Bike:** Flat interval 5 x 5 – this will be riding flat out so at around 80–90 percent of your maximal heart rate for 5 minutes with a 90-second recovery, repeated five times, with a 10-minute warm-up and cool-down ride at an easy pace. This session could also been done as a turbo or spinning bike session.

>>> **Swim:** 200m warm up at an easy pace in any stroke, then rest for 30 seconds; 4 x 25m working at 8–9/10 RPE with a 30-second rest between each 25m in competition stroke, followed by an easy pace for 200m; 8 x 25m working at 8–9/10 RPE with a 15-second recovery between 25m in competition stroke. Repeat this whole sequence three times.

FUEL REQUIREMENTS

These high-intensity training sessions need carbohydrate. You will be unable to do this type of session without it in your system. For females the daily requirement of carbohydrate will be as high as 5g/kg BW if it's an isolated session or 7g/kg BW if you're training twice that day. For males it will be 7g/kg BW if it's an isolated session and as much as 10g/kg BW if you're training twice that day. This equates to 5–9 fist-size portions of carbohydrate distributed throughout the day as meals and snacks. You will also need 5–8 palm-size portions or 0.25g/kg BW protein.

If you are planning to do this session in the morning, pay attention to consuming carbohydrate in your main meal the night before, aiming for 1–2g/kg BW as a serving size. Follow this with a similar portion at breakfast at least 1–2 hours before you plan to train.

If you are planning to do this type of session in the evening, ensure you consume 1g/kg BW carbohydrate at breakfast, lunch and as a pre-training snack prior to the session.

Look at the high-intensity sample menus in Chapter 2 to see how you can ensure you meet your fuel needs, depending on when you are training.

After such a hard session, recovery is going to be important, as previously highlighted in Chapter 2. If you have a session within 12 hours, ensure recovery is within 30 minutes of finishing this session and includes 1.2g/kg BW carbohydrate and 0.25g/kg BW protein in a liquid form with fast-acting carbohydrate and easily digestible protein. A good option is flavoured milk or a Mocha Shake (see page 277).

If your next training session is over 12 hours, ensure recovery is within 2 hours of finishing this session and includes 1.2g/kg BW carbohydrate and 0.25g/kg BW protein as a meal. A good option is Fruity Steak Stir-Fry (see page 233).

> **Tip** *When juggling your training around work, always ensure that you are organized and pre-pack portable options that you can keep in your kit bag.*

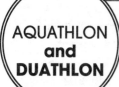

AQUATHLON and DUATHLON

These are modified triathlons, with the aquathlon including only running and swimming while the duathlon comprises cycling and running. The official distances for the Aquathlon World Championships are 2.5K run, 1K swim, and 2.5K run. A duathlon can be contested on almost any terrain, although usually on tarmac. The Duathlon World Championships are held annually and consist of a 10K run, 40K cycle and 5K run.

MULTIPLE SPRINT SPORTS

Multiple sprint sports include activities such as tennis and team sports such as netball, football and basketball. These sports are dependent on both anaerobic and aerobic energy systems (see page 54). Let's look at three specific examples:

>>> **Netball** is a fast-paced, highly skilled sport, which puts considerable demands upon the anaerobic energy systems, with aerobic fitness assisting recovery between bursts of play.

>>> **Football** is an intermittent game involving bursts of high-intensity anaerobic activity, including sprinting, kicking, turning and tackling within an endurance framework.

>>> **Tennis** is a game of skill, speed, agility and concentration, highly reliant on anaerobic energy systems again within an endurance frame. A developed aerobic capacity is advantageous for recovery between points, stamina and tolerance to heat.

A weekly training schedule will include several different sessions to help you as an athlete to adapt to the demands of your sport. There will be skills and technical sessions, strength sessions using weights to develop anaerobic power, game play and also conditioning sessions, building on aerobic fitness and endurance. Each session will have different nutritional demands depending on the overall time, intensity and type of session.

In Chapter 2 we looked at RPE (Rate of Perceived Exertion) to help you train at the right intensities and fuel these sessions appropriately. This is a very relevant method of assessing your needs in these multi-sprint based sports. Table 3.10 below shows the RPE scale and Table 3.11 shows a typical multi-sprint sport training schedule.

Intensity	How this feels	RPE
Easy	Relaxed, easy	5/10
Moderate	Comfortable, controlled	6–7/10
High	Challenging and becoming harder as the session progresses	8–9/10

TABLE 3.10 The RPE scale

Day of the week	Training intensity
Monday	1-hour skills session followed by 1-hour game play
Tuesday	60–90-mins strength session
Wednesday	2-hour game/match play
Thursday	Rest/active recovery
Friday	45-mins conditioning followed by 45 mins strength
Saturday	Competition or 1-hour conditioning followed by 90-mins game play
Sunday	Rest

TABLE 3.11 A typical training week

Now let's look at some examples of actual training sessions for multi-sprint sports and their nutritional demands.

LOW-INTENSITY TRAINING

Due to the nature of multi-sprint sports, the only low-intensity training sessions are on active recovery days or some skills sessions. Working to RPE (see page 68) will help to identify a low-intensity session. Any session where you are working at an intensity of 5/10 RPE, that feels easy, where you can have a conversation and feel quite energized afterwards, is considered to be a low-intensity training session.

FUEL REQUIREMENTS

A low-intensity easy training session has no fuel demands as long as it is kept to a maximum of 60 minutes. A great time to do these sessions is first thing in the morning in a fasted state as your body will obtain what it needs from your fat or glycogen stores. That said, these easy, low-intensity sessions can be done at any time that works for you but there is no need for any specific fuelling strategy in preparation.

So on a day when you are doing an easy pace, low-intensity session or on a rest day, your maximum carbohydrate requirement is 3g/kg BW and your protein requirement is 3–4 servings of 0.25g/kg BW a day. This can be easily achieved by sticking to three meals a day, combining fist-size portions of complex carbohydrate, such as oats, sweet potato, root vegetables or pulses, with a palm-size portion of protein, such as eggs, chicken or fish, served with unlimited undressed salad or vegetables. Snack on fruit or vegetables.

Remember to start the session hydrated and continue to drink as required throughout. Always choose non-nutritive drinks that don't provide any energy, such as water or squash with no added sugar. If it is particularly warm or you are training indoors, for example with netball or tennis, you may have higher sweat losses and these need to be matched to help prevent dehydration, which we know leads to lapses in concentration.

Take some time to refer back to the low-intensity sample menus in Chapter 2. These are really helpful in demonstrating how to meet the nutritional requirements for low-intensity training and rest days. They incorporate recipes from this book, which are suitable to serve up to the whole family while still making sure you meet your training needs.

MODERATE-INTENSITY TRAINING

Moderate-intensity training will feel like you are holding a comfortable pace, working at 6–7/10 on the RPE scale. Some scenarios include:

>>> **Netball:** this will be position dependent but for some players on the team a moderate-intensity session will include match play practice. Always be guided by RPE. Some strength and conditioning sessions will also be moderate intensity:
>> Steady state run or bike sessions
>> Plyometrics (see page 102)

A single game of netball does not place huge nutritional demands on trained athletes. However, the accumulation of regular training sessions and games throughout the week is challenging with regards to recovery, especially if you are juggling training and competing with jobs, study and family commitments. Aim to be as organized as possible, knowing your daily training schedule. Make appropriate nutritional choices around these training sessions, keeping suitable options in your kit bag. Some good examples are:

>>> Long-life tetra packs of flavoured milk – good for recovery

>>> Packets of dried fruit and nuts – watch portion size but these are great as a snack to help control blood sugars and prevent energy dips through the day

>>> Malt loaf to top up stores if you are travelling from work straight to training

>>> Sandwiches, wraps, salads and soups are all good lunch options if you are training or competing later in the evening (see Light Meals, page 197)

Often netball training sessions are scheduled for late in the evening, which requires careful meal planning during the day. If you want to stick with the tradition of having your main meal at night, have it prepared before training so that it can be ready within minutes of arriving home. Although it is important to refuel and recover after exercise, many people feel uncomfortable going to sleep on a very full stomach. An alternative is to restructure the day to make lunch the main meal, and then refuel after the session with a lighter meal or snack before bed. This is where having a small 250ml/9fl oz carton of flavoured milk in the car on the way home is ideal; it starts the recovery process and then you can top up with some toast or a bowl of cereal when you get in.

>>> **Football**: As with netball, this will be dependent on position so for some players a moderate-intensity training session will be match play practice and certain strength and conditioning sessions. Always be guided by your RPE, aiming for 6–7/10.

>>> **Tennis**: Most of you who play tennis will split your week between high-intensity training sessions and strength and conditioning sessions; it is likely that a high percentage of your high-intensity training sessions will be of moderate intensity. Indeed some of your actual competition/match play will end up being moderate intensity, depending on your opponent. Think about your RPE and time on court, and fuel accordingly.

FUEL REQUIREMENTS

These sessions are harder than low-intensity easy sessions but you should still feel within your comfort zone. Your daily carbohydrate requirement will be a maximum of 5g/kg BW and your protein requirement will be 0.25g/kg BW four times a day. The moderate-intensity sample menu plans in Chapter 2 demonstrate what these requirements look like practically and also take into account the time of day you train.

Due to multi-sprint sports being competitive and played against an opposition, fuelling can be tricky. On the one hand it could be an easy match with low fuel demands or the opposite could be true. In tennis fuel requirements may depend on how long you are on court and so appropriate snacks may need to be consumed during the match.

Aim for 1g/kg BW carbohydrate and 0.25g/kg BW protein prior to these sessions, adjusting your intake as needed. So if your session actually turns out to be a tough one with an RPE of 8–9/10 then you will need to increase your carbohydrate intake and consider taking some fuel on during your training. Some good examples include:

>>> Banana

>>> 1–2 pieces of malt loaf

>>> 500ml/17fl oz energy drink – homemade (see page 80) or branded

>>> Dried fruit, such as small boxes of raisins or dates

>>> 5–6 jelly babies

If the session is a lot easier than you anticipated so nearer to an RPE of 6/10, you will need to reduce the amount of carbohydrate in your recovery phase to 0.5g/kg BW, keeping protein at 0.25g/kg BW.

If your session has been of moderate intensity, your recovery needs are 1g/kg BW carbohydrate and 0.25g/kg BW protein. If this is your only training session for the day, aim to eat this recovery meal or snack within 2 hours of completing your session. This may fall at your next meal.

If you are planning to do a second training session within the next 12 hours and your next meal is not imminent after this session, you will need a recovery choice such as the Recovery Hot Chocolate (see page 277) within 30 minutes and followed by a meal 2 hours later.

HIGH-INTENSITY TRAINING

These training sessions are challenging and feel hard with an RPE of 8–9/10. As already mentioned, multi-sprint sports, such as netball, football and tennis, have a high anaerobic demand, working a lot of the time above your lactate threshold. During competition these are displayed as high-speed sprints with more aerobic base work for recovery between. A footballer will sprint (anaerobic) to receive or chase the ball; once he has passed the ball, he will reduce his speed (aerobic) to follow the ball until he is called upon again to receive the ball. So match play will more than likely be a high-intensity session, but there will also be certain conditioning sessions that are done at a high intensity to help develop your aerobic fitness further:

>>> 30–40 minute watt/spin bike session

>>> 45–60 minute run intervals

>>> 30–40 minutes repeated sprints on court with change of direction

FUEL REQUIREMENTS

You will be unable to do this type of high-intensity session without carbohydrate in your system. Your daily requirement of carbohydrate will be as high as 5g/kg BW in females and 7g/kg BW in males, so 5–7 fist-size portions of carbohydrate distributed throughout the day as meals and snacks. Some examples are:

>>> 50g/1$^3/_4$ oz rolled oats

>>> Banana

>>> Fist-size portion of sweet potato

>>> 3–4 oatcakes

>>> Fist-size portion of cooked rice/couscous

>>> Piece of toast

You will also need 4–6 palm-size portions or 0.25g/kg BW protein. If you are planning to do this session in the morning, pay attention to consuming carbohydrate in your main meal the night before, aiming for 1–2g/kg BW as a serving size. Follow this up with a similar portion at breakfast at least 1–2 hours before you plan to train.

If you are planning to do this type of session in the evening, ensure you consume 1g/kg BW carbohydrate at breakfast, lunch and as a pre-training snack prior to the session. Look at the high-intensity sample menus in Chapter 2 to see how you can ensure you meet your fuel needs, depending on when you are training.

After such a hard session, recovery is going to be important, as previously highlighted in Chapter 2. If you have a session within 12 hours, ensure recovery is within 30 minutes of finishing this session and includes 1.2g/kg BW carbohydrate and 0.25g/kg BW protein in a liquid form with fast-acting carbohydrate and easily digestible protein. A good option is flavoured milk or Mocha Shake (see page 277).

If your next training session is over 12 hours, ensure recovery is within 2 hours of finishing this session and includes 1.2g/kg BW carbohydrate and 0.25g/kg BW protein as a meal. Try Roasted Aubergine and Beef Curry (see page 234).

STRENGTH TRAINING

Those of you doing multi-sprint sports will include a high proportion of strength/resistance training during your week. Strength training is important to these sports as it:

>>> Improves anaerobic fitness

>>> Increases power

>>> Can help with body composition:
>> leaner netball players have a higher vertical jump height

>> footballers with low body-fat levels will have more speed, agility and endurance

>> in tennis low body-fat levels provide competitive advantage with regards to greater power behind shots, greater speed and agility around the court

>>> May be needed to increase overall muscle mass

Protein tends to be the most important fuel in resistance training. The best way to achieve a positive protein balance to help with muscle development and adaptation is to use 'protein pulsing' (see page 26). Protein pulsing encourages the intake of 0.25g/kg BW protein 4–6 times a day to help maintain a positive protein balance. This in turn means that the muscle has a constant supply of protein to utilize in order to recover, repair and build/adapt. With strength/resistance training, it is a good idea to include protein foods an hour before and within 1–2 hours of completing your session. For most athletes 0.25g/kg BW protein is around 20–25g of protein. This equates to:

>>> 3 large eggs

>>> 75g/2½oz (half a 150g/5oz can) tuna

>>> 100g/3½oz salmon fillet

>>> 130g/4½oz cod fillet

>>> 130g/4½oz mackerel fillet

>>> 85g/3oz halibut fillet

>>> 100g/3½oz pilchards in brine

>>> 175g/6oz peeled prawns/shrimp

>>> 200g/7oz tofu

>>> 80g/2¾oz portion of pork loin

>>> 4 pork sausages

>>> 600ml/21fl oz skimmed milk

>>> 200g/7oz cottage cheese

>>> 60g/2oz nuts – any unsalted

>>> 70g/2¼oz crunchy peanut butter/almond butter

>>> 1 x 240g/8½oz (drained weight) can chickpeas/kidney beans

>>> 1 x 400g/14oz can baked beans in tomato sauce

>>> 100g/3½oz dry-weight lentils

>>> 100g/3½oz fillet chicken

>>> 60g/2oz Cheddar/feta/mozzarella

>>> 57g/2oz skimmed milk powder

>>> 25g whey powder

Studies suggest that it is useful to have an easily digestible form of protein in the post-training phase as this is readily taken up into the muscles. Low-fat dairy products such as cottage cheese, fat-free Greek yogurt, milk, flavoured milk or whey protein are all good options.

When an athlete needs to increase overall muscle mass or 'bulk up', there are other considerations to take into account. The nutritional requirements for increasing muscle bulk and strength are for protein to form new muscle tissue, and carbohydrate to fuel the training needed to stimulate this muscle growth. Vitamins and minerals are also beneficial. You will need to increase your intake of energy from nutrient-rich food and drinks, such as milkshakes or fruit smoothies, but this should not be seen as an excuse to fill up on energy-dense, nutrient-poor foods such as high-fat takeaway foods or 'junk food'. Try to increase the frequency of food intake rather than the serving sizes as each meal.

Tip *Instead of having a cheese and ham white baguette and a chocolate bar which will be high non-nutrient dense meal, have a chicken salad granary baguette, followed by fruit and yogurt which will provide you with the same amount of energy but additional value in the form of protein, fibre, calcium and vitamins.*

PLANNING YOUR TRAINING WEEK

Although it is important to fuel each training day according to the type of session, you also need to think about how this all flows together in a week. Table 3.12 shows the nutritional considerations for the typical training week we looked at earlier.

Day of the week	Training session	Nutritional considerations
Monday	1-hour skills session followed by 1-hour game play	2-hour session, not high intensity but due to length of time, important to consume 1g/kg BW carbohydrate before and also to consider recovery.
Tuesday	60–90 mins strength session	Important to include 0.25g/kg BW protein before and after this session. If aim is to increase muscle mass and size, add carbohydrate to both options.
Wednesday	2 hours game/ match play	This has the potential to be high intensity for 2 hours so include carbohydrate in the 24 hours before the session.
Thursday	Rest/active recovery	No nutritional demands – continue with protein pulsing but reduce carbohydrate.
Friday	45 mins conditioning followed by 45 mins strength training	90-min session with high-intensity conditioning, so need to include carbohydrate prior to session. Aim for 1–2g/kg BW carbohydrate and 0.25g/kg BW protein. Remember to recover.
Saturday	Competition or 1-hour conditioning followed by 90 mins game play	This has the potential to be high intensity for 2 hours so include carbohydrate 24 hours before the session.
Sunday	Rest	No nutritional demands – continue with protein pulsing but reduce carbohydrate.

TABLE 3.12 Nutritional Considerations for a typical training week

Nutritional considerations for multiple sprint sports

Due to the nature of these sports, there are further nutritional considerations above those of fuelling demands:

>>> **Off-season:** There will usually be a period of time where training is significantly reduced. It is important to adjust your nutritional intake accordingly. This will help to prevent weight/body composition fluctuations so that you start the new season in good shape.

>>> **Travelling:** A lot of matches and tournaments will be played away from home. Although this is probably some of the appeal of playing this sport, it can also make life quite difficult nutritionally. Trying to find familiar or suitable foods can be tricky and may lead to over- consuming non-nutritive energy-dense foods or not fuelling sufficiently, leading to poor performance. Try to find out as much as you can about where you will be staying so that you can take snacks to supplement your diet.

>>> **Team-based:** Being part of a team is fun and supportive. However, the pressure to perform can also be high as you won't want to let the whole team down. One of the key things is to encourage good practice amongst the team; think about a team pre-match meal or consider nominating someone within the team who can provide appropriate recovery choices. Hydration is also very important. We know that just 2 percent dehydration, 1kg/2.2lb in a 50kg/110lb athlete, can have significant effects on performance but also concentration. These sports have a high skill element; becoming dehydrated can impair the decision-making process severely. It may only affect one member of the team but it will have an impact on everyone. Try to remind each other to drink and stay hydrated.

Summary

>>> Whatever your sport, ensure you are training at the correct intensity to condition the right energy systems

>>> Your training week should include a mixture of low-, moderate- and high-intensity training days

>>> Each level of training intensity requires different nutritional needs

>>> Snacks play an important role in fuelling for and recovering from training, as well as keeping up energy levels throughout

>>> Make sure you plan your fuel around your training, and that you take the right foods with you if there is any doubt that they will be available

>>> Whatever sport you are doing and at whatever level, make sure you are well hydrated at all times

CHAPTER 4:
FINE-TUNING YOUR BODY

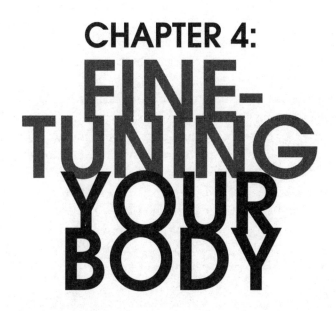

TROUBLESHOOTING COMPLAINTS

The human body is extremely efficient and clever, but it's not perfect. Although participating in sport is important for good health, sport itself is not always beneficial for our bodies. Indeed, rates of injury are usually high in athletes. Whether it is a twisted joint, a pulled muscle/ligament or something more serious, training for a sport puts a huge strain on the body and, inevitably, can lead to injury or overuse.

Nutrition is a continually evolving science, with new studies and research being published on a daily basis. An area that is of real interest to researchers is how nutrition can impact on injury prevention and how recovery from injury can be encouraged using nutrition. As with all studies, there are mixed results and, although further research is required, overall there do seem to be some key nutritional strategies that may be beneficial.

In this chapter we will look at some common issues associated with sport, the stresses they can potentially cause your body and how nutrition can help to restore balance.

COMMON COMPLAINTS

Training is a time-consuming business. Whether you are an elite athlete who needs to commit to over 4 hours training daily or a recreational athlete who is trying to fit training in with work and family commitments, it is inevitable that sometimes you might take shortcuts. Some examples are:

>>> Not warming up sufficiently before training

>>> Not stretching after training

>>> Using poor technique or 'cheating' to get an exercise done quickly

>>> Being disorganized and so having poor nutritional options available around training

These shortcuts may leave your body feeling unbalanced and vulnerable. You may also choose to ignore early symptoms, which can potentially become something more serious further down the line. These symptoms might include:

>>> Pain

>>> Fatigue

>>> Poor sleep patterns

>>> Dizziness

>>> Shortness of breath

>>> Skipping menstruation

In all these cases, addressing the issue early can help to prevent longer-term problems and, in most cases, it is usually quite easy to fix!

INJURY PREVENTION

There are many things you can do to help prevent injury – many athletes are now familiar with the four Rs:

1 > Rehydrate – sweating causes a loss of water and electrolytes, so make sure you drink water before, during and after exercise to avoid dehydration.

2 > Replenish – stored carbohydrate (glycogen) is the primary fuel for muscles during exercise. It is important to consume carbohydrate after exercise to replace depleted stores, but be guided by the intensity of your training session. See Chapters 2 and 3.

3 > Repair – muscle is broken down during exercise – eating high-quality protein after exercise will help to rebuild muscle tissue.

4 > Reinforce – during exercise your immune system becomes compromised due to cell damage and inflammation. To keep a strong immune system, you should refuel with nutritious, fresh foods.

Tip *Personally I also think there is a fifth R – Rest. We will look at this with overtraining later in this chapter.*

So from the above we can see that nutrition plays a huge part in injury prevention. Helping your body to stay in alignment and strengthening potential weak areas within the body will also be useful.

USING MUSCLES CORRECTLY

Moving correctly is a skill. Throughout life and our sporting endeavours, we often develop bad habits or 'cheats', where we have a tendency to move incorrectly to shortcut a result and to compensate in a way that leads to bad posture, muscle imbalances and incorrect co-ordination of muscles. The human body is designed to use different muscles for different tasks. This is why we have:

>>> Big, bulky muscles for producing large forces

>>> Long, thin muscles for supporting bones in the correct position for long durations

>>> Different-shaped muscles to move the joints at the correct angles

Ideally we use our deep, small, stabilizing muscles to hold our posture and keep joints in the correct alignment, while the superficial big muscles are responsible for contracting and relaxing in sequence to produce major movements.

In order for this to happen we must have a good technique for our training movements and our sport-specific movements, and we must train our 'stabilizing' muscles to stabilize and our 'moving' muscles to move the joints and limbs. Problems occur when we neglect one or the other and end up using movers to stabilize – for example, using the

hip flexors to support the torso rather than the deep
and glutes, or using the pectoral muscles to support †
rather than the rotator cuff. This means that the mo
available for their primary role – moving – and it c
bones to be pulled slightly out of alignment lead
joints, weak links and subsequent irritation, ⌐

To train the stabilizers you need progressive movements ⌐
For example, a typical progression would be floor-based core exercises
such as Pilates; once core strength has been established, you would
progress to a standing single leg squat, using the stabilizers to keep the
joints in alignment while the movers execute the squat itself. The final
progression would be to execute a sports skill at full speed and intensity
or a maximal or explosive strength exercise with good posture and joint
alignment. So let's take running as an example – most runners tend to
use their hamstrings rather than their glutes to produce movement, often
leading to hamstring injuries such as tendinopathy. By using the above
progression example, you will be able to engage your glutes more when
you are out running, preventing injury but also improving performance.

NUTRITION FOR SORE, TIRED OR INJURED BODIES

One way to help avoid injury is to organize your nutrition
around your training so that you are meeting your requirements.
Hopefully by now, having read through this book so far, you will
have a real understanding of how to do that but there are some
further nutritional strategies you may find useful. This is a huge
area of growth with regards to researching how specific nutrients
can aid the body to return to an optimal state prior to the next
training session.

DOMS, or delayed onset muscle soreness, is a common phenomenon in athletes, especially those who have taken on a new form of training – such as adding strength to weekly cycling mileage – or those who have trained or competed particularly hard. The soreness is most commonly felt 24–72 hours after the exercise. This is due to micro-trauma, which is mechanical damage at a very small scale to the muscles being exercised, leading to inflammation and oxidative stress. Oxidative stress is the term used to describe the damage to proteins, membranes and genes by free radicals. Studies have shown that although exercise is good for us, it does also increase the amount of free radicals in our body.

Usually if you repeat this exercise pattern sufficiently, your body will get used to it and the soreness will stop. However, we also know that to improve performance, muscles need to be 'overloaded' continually and so DOMS will be inevitable from time to time.

There has been a lot of research into this area to help with reducing inflammation and oxidative stress, with the best findings coming from the use of powerful antioxidants such as:

>>> Curcumin – found in cumin

>>> Isoflavanoids – found in soya beans

>>> Polyphenols – most of the data has come from studies using tart cherry juice, which did seem to show a significant reduction in inflammatory markers in endurance athletes after strenuous sessions

>>> Vitamin C

However, in all these cases, further studies were needed to help decide on dose and timings for optimal benefits. That said, I actively encourage individuals to increase their intake of antioxidants through food by consuming more fruit, vegetables, herbs and spices (see the Nepalese Chicken Curry recipe on page 288 for one of many spicy recipes). They are important providers of vitamins and minerals but also potentially have the benefit of preventing muscle soreness.

INJURED BODY

The most important thing to remember when you are injured is that you need to rest. Depending on the severity of your injury, you may need as little as a few days to as long as 3 months. Being injured is very frustrating, especially when training has been going well. However, it is also a good time to reflect and work out how you will prevent this from becoming a problem again:

>>> Did you ignore signs of pain?

>>> Did you fuel and recover appropriately after training?

>>> Did you take sufficient rest between sessions?

>>> Do you need to look at the way in which you use your body and start to include some strength and stabilizing work (see page 96)?

Nutrition can also be instrumental in your recovery and return to exercise. A lot of athletes understandably worry about weight gain when they become injured. Research has demonstrated that by decreasing your overall energy intake but increasing your protein intake to as high as 2.3g/kg BW daily is useful. Firstly, protein has a high satiety factor so it helps you to feel full while limiting your overall energy intake and, secondly, the protein itself has been shown to help with actual repair of the damaged area. Similarly, if you have a bone injury, such as a stress fracture, supplementing with vitamin D has been shown to be effective (see below).

••

VITAMIN D

Vitamin D is a fat-soluble vitamin that functions as a hormone. Its structure is similar to steroid hormones such as oestrogen and testosterone. There has been a lot of interest in vitamin D over the last few years. It has always been known for its role in preserving bone health but it has now also been linked to many other aspects of health and optimal muscle function.

We make vitamin D in our bodies from sunlight. However, those who live in countries where sunlight might be limited, those who spend little time outdoors, those who cover up with high-factor sunscreen and those who are darker-skinned, may actually be at risk of a vitamin D deficiency. A vitamin D deficiency can lead to several health issues such as:

>>> Chronic fatigue

>>> Depression

>>> Increased risk of bone injury

>>> Chronic musculoskeletal pain

>>> Viral respiratory tract infections

There also seems to be emerging strong evidence that supplementing an athlete who has sub-optimal levels of vitamin D has real benefits to performance, particularly in strength, power, reaction time and balance.

There is no universally accepted definition for vitamin D deficiency but the following classifications from blood test levels are often cited:

>>> When blood levels are below 50nmol/L – deficiency

>>> When blood levels are below 75nmol/L – insufficient levels

>>> Increased risk of bone injury

>>> Levels between 75–120nmol/L – ideal range

Vitamin D supplements are readily available but if you are an athlete, always make sure that you buy from a reputable source.

You will not be able to meet your requirements through food alone but small amounts of vitamin D can be found in the following foods:

>>> Oily fish

>>> Egg yolks

>>> Fortified foods such as milk, margarine and cereals

• •

TIRED BODY

When you are training hard, you are bound to feel a residual amount of fatigue. However, if tiredness does not disappear after a few days' rest, it is important to take note and consider what else could be contributing.

Some questions to ask yourself:

>>> Have I increased or changed my training significantly recently?

>>> Am I taking enough rest or active recovery time between hard or long sessions?

>>> Am I recovering appropriately nutritionally?

>>> Am I hydrated?

>>> Am I eating enough before I train?

>>> Is it possible I am coming down with a virus or illness?

If the answer to all the above is no, ask yourself whether you have any other symptoms?

Tiredness can be the first sign of iron-deficiency anaemia, especially if coupled with some of the other symptoms such as dizziness, shortness of breath, pale skin colour, blue-tinged dark circles around the eyes, poor appetite and a reduction in athletic performance. For more information on iron and how to include it in your diet, see Chapter 1.

OVERTRAINING

As athletes we often push ourselves with the sole aim of improving our performance to meet our specific goals. This is not a problem as long as you learn to listen to your body, resting when it needs to and fuelling appropriately. However, sometimes things can get out of balance; we choose not to rest or recover adequately between sessions, which can present itself in many ways but always ends with poor performance outcomes.

Overtraining syndrome, or OTS, can best be defined as the state where an athlete has been repeatedly stressed by training to the point where rest is no longer adequate to allow for recovery. The 'overtraining syndrome' is the name given to the collection of emotional, behavioural, and physical symptoms due to overtraining that has persisted for weeks to months. This is different from the day-to-day variation in performance and post-exercise tiredness that is common in conditioned athletes. Overtraining is marked by cumulative exhaustion that persists even after recovery periods. Some common features to be aware of include:

>>> Lack of energy

>>> Mild leg soreness, general aches and pains

>>> Pain in muscles and joints

>>> Sudden drop in performance

>>> Insomnia

>>> Headaches

>>> Decrease in immunity, leading to more colds and sore throats

>>> Decrease in training capacity / intensity

>>> Moodiness and irritability

>>> Depression/low mood

>>> Loss of enthusiasm for the sport

>>> Decreased appetite

>>> Increased incidence of injuries

>>> A compulsive need to exercise

It can sometimes be difficult to distinguish overtraining, as you may not exhibit all of the symptoms mentioned above. That said, there are several ways you can objectively measure it. One such method includes documenting your heart rate at specific training intensities and speeds over a period of time. If your pace at a given intensity starts to slow but your heart rate is increased or your resting heart rate increases, or the perceived effort of doing an easy session is consistently higher than it should be, you may be heading into overtraining syndrome.

> **Tip**
>
> *Take your pulse each morning before getting out of bed. If there is a marked increase, 10 beats per minute higher than normal, this may indicate that you aren't fully recovered and should take an extra day or more to recover. The amount of time you need to recover will depend on the length of time you have been overtraining.*

Research on OTS shows that getting adequate rest is the most important thing. Total recovery from overtraining can take several weeks and should include reducing stress and proper nutrition, including complex carbohydrates, lean protein, fruits and vegetables and staying hydrated. Try the delicious smoothies and salads in the recipe section.

DISEQUILIBRIUM AND THE POTENTIAL PROBLEMS

Sometimes training and nutrition can become unbalanced. OTS is one example of how the body can react to this but there are other potential problems that can occur if good nutrition and rest do not make up an integral part of your training programme.

When we are training hard, sometimes it is difficult to detect if we are getting sufficient amounts of energy to meet our day-to-day needs as well as our increased exercise demands. In general terms if you listen to your body, and fuel as required for your chosen activity and intensity, equilibrium can be maintained. However in some cases, energy demands of training can be a challenge to meet. For some this will result in weight loss, which may or may not be wanted and which needs to be addressed accordingly. Sometimes it is not so clear-cut. There are occasions when weight stays stable but available energy is low; energy intake is not sufficient to meet daily requirements, whether this is due to a conscious decision to restrict nutritional intake (disequilibrium is sometimes due to an eating disorder) or simply an inability to meet the demands of training. When energy availability is low the body preserves energy by deeming the reproductive system as not essential, therefore lowering the level of sex hormones in the body. This is easy to detect in females as it usually represents itself as a missed period; it is much harder to detect in males. In both cases this is not an ideal situation and needs to be addressed.

We have already looked at the importance of vitamin D and calcium (see pages 28 and 171) for bone health. However, a lot of people are not aware that having low energy availability can also lead to significant decreases in bone density and overall bone health. In the female athlete, missing three consecutive periods can have potentially negative effects on bone health; it can take as long as 6 months of regular menstruation to reverse this damage.

Similarly if body-fat levels drop too low in athletes, this will also have a negative effect on bone density. In female athletes, dropping to a body fat of 12 percent or below will once again suppress sex hormones and cease menstruation. In male athletes, a level of 6 percent or below will have a negative effect on bone health, in particular bone density. Dexa scans can be used to measure bone density. A low level is used to diagnose osteoporosis, which is a potentially serious condition where compromised bone strength may predispose someone to an increased risk of fractures.

As mentioned, it is difficult to detect problems in male athletes but some symptoms to look for in both genders that demonstrate low body-fat levels or poor energy availability include:

>>> Feeling extremes in temperature, both hot and cold, due to low body-fat levels and being unable to regulate heat

>>> Feeling dizzy or disorientated due to low blood glucose

>>> Poor/low libido

>>> Poor concentration

>>> Poor sleep patterns

>>> Recurrent stress fractures

>>> Irritability

>>> Poor recovery between sessions and reduced performance

>>> Withdrawal from social circle and situations

By restoring energy availability, it is possible to reverse the effect on bone health in the following ways. Adequate energy availability promotes bone health:

>>> *Directly* by stimulating the production of hormones that promote bone formation

>>> *Indirectly* by preserving menstruation and oestrogen production that stems bone resorption

In most cases it is simply a case of addressing these energy needs and providing nutritional advice that will encourage a minimum of 30Kcals/kg BW of fat-free mass. I always encourage individuals who have had an episode where energy availability has been low to increase their intake of calcium to 1,600mg a day, which is four servings of dairy, and also take a high-dose vitamin D supplement (see page 172) to aid the recovery process.

However, sometimes it is not quite as simple. If the individual has developed irregular eating patterns or is suffering from an eating disorder, this is a lot more difficult to reverse. It can take months and involves a multi-disciplinary team approach with a registered dietitian/nutritionist, psychologist, coach, if there is one available, and a GP or other doctor.

....

THE FEMALE HORMONE CYCLE

The menstrual cycle can have a real influence on a female athlete's energy levels and energy intake. During the follicular phase, days 1–13, where day 1 is the first day of your period, oestrogen levels are rising and peak just before ovulation (days 14/15), while progesterone levels are low. During the luteal phase, days 16–28, oestrogen levels decrease, falling to the lowest level just before your period starts; progesterone is at its highest point midway through this luteal phase. These hormones control what type of fuel you oxidize/utilize.

It has been well documented that when oestrogen levels are high, that is just before you ovulate, women use a higher percentage of fat for energy. As oestrogen levels drop and progesterone levels rise, our bodies become more dependent on carbohydrate for fuel, which explains the sugar cravings most women experience just before their period. Additionally, high progesterone levels are linked to an increase in protein catabolism, the breakdown of proteins.

These changes in levels of oestrogen and progesterone also influence temperature change within the body; most women find that a reduction in oestrogen and increase in progesterone during the luteal phase causes a rise in temperature. How many of you that are not near post-menopausal age have woken up with night sweats and wondered what this is about? Now you know! This increase in temperature is also linked to a small increase in overall energy expenditure, which helps to explain the increased hunger and appetite we also feel during this time.

From a nutritional point of view, I suggest that in the 7–10 days prior to your period, so during the luteal phase of your menstrual cycle, you make small dietary changes. Aim to include small frequent snacks of both complex carbohydrate and protein every 2–3 hours to prevent blood-sugar fluctuations. Some good examples include:

>>> Fat-free Greek yogurt with fruit and honey

>>> Hot chocolate made with milk (see Recovery Hot Chocolate, page 277)

>>> Wholegrain toast with Nut Butter (see page 191)

>>> Eggs on toast

>>> Dried fruit and nuts

>>> Oatcakes with cheese

As we have already seen, the levels of hormones during your menstrual cycle can influence the types of fuel you will use for energy. This has a significant impact during ultra distance events. During such events your body will ultimately run out of glycogen and thus readily available glucose stores within a couple of hours; it will look for other means to provide energy for the working muscles. This could be via fuel you take on during your event – or gluconeogenesis is a further potential pathway for this. Gluconeogenesis is a method by which the body breaks down non-carbohydrate sources of fuel into glucose. The most common of these sources within the body will be fatty acids from fat stores and amino acids from muscle.

However at certain points of your menstrual cycle; namely just after ovulation and at the start of the luteal phase (ie when both oestrogen and progesterone levels are equal), gluconeogenesis is suppressed. This suppression means that in order to continue to meet your fuel requirements for the duration of your ultra distance event, you will need to take on sufficient amounts of carbohydrate; 90g of carbohydrate per hour has been quoted as the optimal amount needed.

Summary

>>> Nutrition can play an important role in injury prevention and healing – you are less likely to suffer injuries if you are well nourished, and will heal more quickly if you do

>>> Antioxidants, such as those found in herbs and spices or fruit and vegetables, can play a role in reducing inflammation and soreness of muscles

>>> When injured, a combination of rest and an increased intake of protein are the keys to the body repairing itself

>>> Not allowing the body to recover adequately between training sessions is a symptom of Overtraining Syndrome

>>> Not consuming enough of the correct foods can lead to disequilibrium, so it is important to make sure energy demands are being met

>>> Small dietary changes can help balance female hormones during the menstrual cycle, and minimize its impact on training

BREAKFASTS

Breakfast Shake

This makes a great on-the-go breakfast, or is perfect for recovery after an early-morning training session.

Serves 1   **Preparation time:** 5 minutes

125g/4½oz/½ cup low-fat fruit yogurt, any flavour
200ml/7fl oz/¾ cup skimmed milk
30g/1oz/heaped ¼ cup rolled oats
1 tbsp clear honey

1 Put all the ingredients in a blender and blend until smooth. Serve straight away.

Nutrition facts (per smoothie)   Calories 344   Carbohydrate 60g
Protein 16g   Fat 3.5g (of which saturates 0g)

Summer Fruit Smoothie

A refreshing pre-workout smoothie full of summer berries, which are known for their vaso-dilation properties, encouraging more oxygen uptake to working muscles.

Serves 1   **Preparation time:** 5 minutes

10 raspberries
5 strawberries
1 tbsp redcurrants
100g/3½oz/⅓ cup fat-free Greek yogurt
1 handful of ice
100ml/3½fl oz/⅓ cup skimmed milk

1 Put all the ingredients in a blender and blend until smooth. Serve straight away.

Nutrition facts (per smoothie)   Calories 183   Carbohydrate 36g
Protein 10g   Fat 0g (of which saturates 0g)

Cranberry & Mango Smoothie

This lovely, refreshing smoothie could be used as a pre- or post-training option. If you prefer to choose this as a recovery option, substitute the plain yogurt for fat-free Greek yogurt as it has a much higher percentage of protein, which is necessary for the repair of cells.

Serves 1   **Preparation time:** 5 minutes

½ ripe mango, peeled, pitted and roughly chopped
250ml/9fl oz/1 cup cranberry juice
125g/4oz/½ cup fat-free plain yogurt

1 Put the mango and cranberry juice in a blender and blend for 1 minute. Add the yogurt and blend until smooth. Serve straight away.

Nutrition facts (per smoothie) Calories 244 Carbohydrate 46g
Protein 9g Fat 2.9g (of which saturates 1.5g)

Banana & Almond Smoothie

This is an ideal recovery smoothie for breakfast or for any time. The combination of ingredients makes it a good source of fast-release carbohydrate and protein in a ratio of 3:1. This will enhance glycogen re-synthesis and repair muscles after training. If you don't have a banana in the freezer, add a handful of ice instead.

Serves 1   **Preparation time:** 5 minutes

1 ripe banana, frozen
250ml/9fl oz/1 cup skimmed milk
2 tsp Nut Butter (see page 191) made with almonds

1 Peel and chop the banana, then put it in a blender with the remaining ingredients. Blend until smooth. Serve straight away.

Nutrition facts (per smoothie) Calories 259 Carbohydrate 42g
Protein 11g Fat 6g (of which saturates 0.5g)

Granola Pot

This is another great portable breakfast that can be eaten at your desk. It is high in carbohydrate, and adding some fat-free Greek yogurt also turns it into a great choice for recovery. If you make a larger quantity of the Granola, you can store it in an airtight container for a week or so. Then you can prepare your Granola Pot the night before you want it, pop it in the fridge, and you are good to go in the morning.

Serves 1   **Preparation time:** 5 minutes   **Cooking time:** 15 minutes

For the Granola (makes 10 servings):
100g/3½oz/¾ cup sunflower seeds
300g/10½oz/3 cups rolled oats
200g/7oz/2¼ cups flaked/slivered almonds
100ml/3½fl oz/⅓ cup clear honey
100g/3½oz/1¼ cups coconut flakes

300g/10½oz/2½ cups dried cherries or other dried fruit of your choice

For the Granola Pot:
100g/3½oz Granola
150g/5½oz/generous ½ cup fat-free Greek yogurt

1 First, make the Granola. Preheat the oven to 150°C/300°F/Gas 2. Put the sunflower seeds, rolled oats and almonds on a baking sheet and drizzle the honey evenly over the top. Bake for 10–15 minutes until golden.

2 Leave the mixture to cool, then stir in the coconut flakes and dried fruit. Store in an airtight container.

3 To make the Granola Pot, take one serving of Granola and put half in a suitable container. Top with the yogurt, then add the remaining mixture. Store in the fridge ready for the next morning or serve straight away.

Nutrition facts (per serving)   Calories 479   Carbohydrate 52g   Protein 26g   Fat 16.9g (of which saturates 4.3g)

Blueberry Bircher Muesli

This is one of my all-time favourite breakfasts, especially in the summer months after an easy early morning run with my spaniel, Bailey. The complex carbohydrate from the oats combined with the high protein from the Greek yogurt mean that this breakfast provides me with slow-release energy all the way through to lunch.

Serves 1   **Preparation time:** 5 minutes, plus overnight soaking

For the Blueberry Compôte (makes 4 servings):
350g/12oz/2½ cups blueberries

For the Bircher Muesli:
85g/3oz Blueberry Compôte
30g /1oz/heaped ¼ cup rolled oats
170g/6oz/heaped ⅔ cup fat-free Greek yogurt
2 tsp clear honey

1 Put the blueberries in a saucepan with 4 tablespoons water over a medium heat. Bring to the boil, then turn the heat down to low and simmer for about 10 minutes until the blueberries are soft and slightly thickened.

2 Leave the compôte to cool, then transfer to a screw-topped jar and keep in the fridge for up to 3 days.

3 To make the Muesli, put a quarter of the Blueberry Compôte (85g/3oz) in a bowl, stir in the oats, cover and leave to soak in the fridge overnight.

4 Stir in the yogurt and honey and enjoy.

Nutrition facts (per serving)   Calories 291   Carbohydrate 52.2g
Protein 17.3g   Fat 2.5g (of which saturates 0g)

Black Forest Porridge

This is an indulgent porridge/oatmeal originally designed for special occasions like Christmas and Easter, but there is nothing stopping you from having this on a race-day morning! Just remember to try it out beforehand as it is not like any porridge/oatmeal you have tasted before, and you want to ensure it won't cause stomach upsets.

Serves 1   **Preparation time:** 5 minutes   **Cooking time:** 5 minutes

55g/2oz/heaped ½ cup rolled oats
200ml/7fl oz/¾ cup skimmed milk
25g/1oz dark/bittersweet chocolate (at least 70% cocoa solids), chopped
30g/¼ cup dried cherries

1 **Put the oats, milk and chocolate in a saucepan over a low heat for 3–5 minutes, stirring occasionally, until the chocolate has melted, all the milk has been absorbed and the porridge is thick.**

2 **Transfer to a bowl, stir in the cherries and serve hot.**

Nutrition facts (per serving) Calories 468 Carbohydrate 73.4g Protein 15.6g Fat 12.1g (of which saturates 6.5g)

HERO FOOD: MILK

It has been well documented that milk is the ideal choice for recovery from high-intensity exercise. When you look at the recommendations for recovery in terms of carbohydrate and protein, the suggested amounts are equal to a 3:1 ratio of carbohydrate to protein. This ratio ensures ideal recovery for the body, particularly after high-intensity exercise, training or competition, when glycogen stores will be completely or close to completely depleted. This is further enhanced if carbohydrate is in a fast release form and protein is easily digestible. The milk sugar (lactose) and whey protein in milk provide this balance, making it a perfect recovery choice. Additionally, milk is a good source of minerals and electrolytes, which are also important for rehydrating post exercise.

Cinnamon Apple Porridge

This warming breakfast is ideal before going out for a run on a cold, frosty morning. Packed with slow-release carbohydrate from the oats, the mixed spice adds a touch of warmth, while the antioxidants it contains give your immune system a boost to ward off colds and infections during the colder months of the year.

Serves 1   **Preparation time:** 5 minutes   **Cooking time:** 1 minute

1 eating apple, such as Cox's, peeled, cored and chopped
¼ tsp mixed/apple pie spice
55g/2oz/heaped ½ cup rolled oats
200ml/7fl oz/¾ cup skimmed milk
30g/1oz/¼ cup raisins

1 Put the apple and spice in a saucepan with 3 tablespoons water over a medium heat. Bring to the boil, then turn the heat down to low and simmer for about 5 minutes, stirring occasionally, until soft.

2 Put the oats and milk in another saucepan over a low heat, bring to the boil, then simmer for 3–5 minutes, stirring occasionally, until the milk has been absorbed and the porridge/oatmeal is thick.

3 Transfer to a bowl, stir in the spiced apple and raisins and serve hot.

Nutrition facts (per serving) Calories 446 Carbohydrate 93g
Protein 15.2g Fat 3.8g (of which saturates 0.7g)

Sunflower Seed & Chia Porridge

This is a real nutrient-packed breakfast. With the nuts boosting its protein and essential fat content, it is a sound choice for before long endurance-training sessions or after training as a recovery option. Using milk, rather than water, will make a creamier, heavier porridge/oatmeal, which is better for recovery.

Serves 1   **Preparation time:** 5 minutes   **Cooking time:** 5 minutes

2 tsp sunflower seeds
55g/2oz/heaped ½ cup rolled oats
200ml/7fl oz/¾ cup skimmed milk or water
1 tsp chia seeds
2 tsp ground almonds
a drizzle of clear honey

1 Put the sunflower seeds in a dry saucepan over a medium heat and toss for a few minutes until just beginning to brown.

2 Add the oats, milk, chia seeds and ground almonds, bring to the boil, then turn the heat down to low and simmer for 3–5 minutes, stirring occasionally, until the milk has been absorbed and the porridge/oatmeal is thick.

3 Transfer to a bowl, stir in the honey to taste and serve hot.

Nutrition facts (per serving) Calories 403 Carbohydrate 56g Protein 18g Fat 11.3g (of which saturates 1.4g)

Apple Breakfast Bread

There is no longer an excuse to not eat breakfast. Whether you claim to be just 'not a breakfast' person or leave the house very early, this bread is easy to prepare in advance and provides a nutritious breakfast eaten on its own or toasted and topped with honey or Nut Butter (see page 191). It also doubles up as a portable snack to eat either before or during a high-intensity training session.

Makes 8 slices   **Preparation time:** 10 minutes   **Cooking time:** 30 minutes

a little rapeseed/canola oil, for greasing
150g/5½oz/scant 1¼ cups spelt flour
200g/7oz/1⅓ cups wholemeal flour
½ tsp salt
1 tsp bicarbonate of soda/baking soda

1 large or 2 small eating apples, such as Cox's, peeled, cored and coarsely grated
55g/2oz/scant ½ cup walnuts, chopped
60ml/2fl oz/¼ cup walnut oil
2 tbsp clear honey
1 egg
200ml/7fl oz/¾ cup apple juice

1 Preheat the oven to 180°C/350°F/Gas 4 and lightly grease a 450g/1lb loaf pan.

2 Mix together the flours, salt and bicarbonate of soda/baking soda in a bowl, then fold in the grated apple. Reserve 1 tablespoon of the nuts, then stir the rest into the mixture. Gently stir in the walnut oil, honey, egg and apple juice, being careful not to over-mix. Spoon the mixture into the prepared pan and scatter the reserved nuts over the top.

3 Bake for 30 minutes, or until a skewer inserted in the centre comes out clean.

4 Leave to cool in the pan for 10–15 minutes, then turn out and transfer to a wire rack. Serve warm or cold. The loaf will keep in an airtight container for up to 3 days.

Nutrition facts (per slice) Calories 173 Carbohydrate 27.5g Protein 6g Fat 5.2g (of which saturates 0g)

Nut Butter, Honey & Oat Muffins

These make a great breakfast and are especially useful when you are racing away from home as they are also easy to transport. A lot of endurance events start very early in the morning, when nerves and staying in a hotel or camping overnight don't always make it easy to have a cooked breakfast. That's when these nutritious muffins are ideal. They can also be used during an endurance event to top up your carbohydrate intake.

Makes 12 muffins   **Preparation time:** 10 minutes   **Cooking time:** 35 minutes

225g/8oz/1½ cups wholemeal spelt flour
75g/3oz/¾ cup rolled oats
1 tbsp baking powder
2 eggs
100g/3½oz/⅓ cup clear honey

2 bananas, mashed
100g/3½oz Nut Butter of your choice (see page 191)
3 tbsp rapeseed/canola oil
100 ml/3½fl oz/⅓ cup skimmed milk

1 Preheat the oven to 190°C/375°F/Gas 5 and line a 12-hole muffin pan with paper muffin cases.

2 Mix together the flour, oats and baking powder in a large bowl and make a well in the centre.

3 Beat the eggs in another bowl, then gently beat in the honey, mashed bananas, Nut Butter, oil and milk until the mixture is fairly sloppy. Tip the mixture into the dry ingredients and mix together quickly but don't over-mix.

4 Spoon the mixture into the prepared muffin cases and bake for 25–30 minutes until the tops are golden brown.

5 Transfer to a wire rack to cool.

Nutrition facts (per muffin) Calories 165 Carbohydrate 18.1g Protein 4g Fat 9.3g (of which saturates 1g)

Race Day Bagel with Nut Butter

Bagels are packed with carbohydrate, ideal for before an endurance event: 60g carbohydrate from one bagel compared with 30–40g from two slices of toast or 50g/1¾oz rolled oats – and this is topped with a banana. The Nut Butter helps to slow down the carb release and prevent blood-sugar dips. You can buy it from the supermarket or health-food store, but making your own from your favourite nuts just takes a little patience. Walnuts are high in omega-3 fats, so make a nutritious butter that is especially good in savoury dishes, mixed with pesto or used in cake recipes that include walnuts. Almonds are high in calcium so are a great choice for vegans or those who struggle to get enough calcium without dairy options. Brazil nuts are high in the antioxidant selenium, which is necessary for many biological processes within the body.

Serves 1   Preparation time: 35 minutes   Cooking time: 3 minutes

For the Nut Butter (makes 310g/11oz):
310g/11oz/2 cups whole nuts of your
   choice, such as almonds, hazelnuts,
   cashew nuts or walnuts

For the Race Day Bagel:
1 wholemeal bagel
25g/1oz Nut Butter
1 large banana

1 First make the Nut Butter. Put the nuts in a food processor and run the machine for 12–15 minutes, stopping regularly to scrape the nuts down the side of the processor bowl and loosen the mixture from the base. Continue to process until the nuts are finely ground and form a ball around the blade. Keep processing until the nuts release their oil and the mixture forms a soft, smooth butter. Store in an airtight jar in the fridge for up to 3 weeks.

2 Preheat the grill/broiler to high.

3 Slice the bagel in half horizontally and toast the cut sides, then spread them with the Nut Butter. Slice the banana on top and serve straight away.

Nutrition facts (per serving)   Calories 470   Carbohydrate 80g   Protein 18g
Fat 18g (of which saturates 2g)

Scrambled Egg Pitta

This is a powerhouse of a breakfast. Two large eggs provide around 20g protein, which is the recommended amount to consume in the recovery phase after exercise. When stuffed into a wholemeal pitta, you add some complex carbohydrate, making this an effective recovery meal.

Serves 1   **Preparation time:** 5 minutes   **Cooking time:** 5 minutes

2 large eggs
1 tbsp skimmed milk
1 large wholemeal pitta bread
sea salt and freshly ground black pepper
1 tbsp apple chutney, to serve

1 Put the eggs and milk in a bowl and whisk together until fluffy. Season with a little salt and pepper. Pour into a non-stick saucepan over a low heat and cook for 2–3 minutes, stirring continuously, until the eggs have stiffened and come away from the side of the pan.

2 Meanwhile, heat the grill/broiler to high and toast the pitta bread, then slice it open. Spoon the scrambled egg mixture into the pocket of the pitta and serve hot or cold with a spoonful of chutney.

Nutrition facts (per serving) Calories 303 Carbohydrate 30g Protein 19g Fat 10.7g (of which saturates 3.3g)

HERO FOOD: EGGS

They may be small, but eggs really pack a punch when it comes to nutritional value; 2 medium eggs will provide you with around 15g of protein, 100 per cent of your daily requirement of vitamin B12 (essential for the formation of red blood cells) and are also packed with selenium, a powerful antioxidant. A lot of people still avoid eggs due to the concern over cholesterol, but in fact a medium egg only contains 4.6g of fat, of which only 1.3g comes from saturated fat. Studies have also shown that individuals who consumed two eggs for breakfast every morning ate 300 calories less the rest of the day, making eggs a great start to the day on low intensity or rest days!

Poached Egg Muffins with Avocado

This is a staple for me after my long Sunday runs when I'm in full marathon training. Once again, the combination of the protein from the eggs and complex carbohydrate from the wholemeal muffin make it a great choice for a recovery breakfast. Eggs are also a good source of other nutrients such as B vitamins, iron, vitamin D, and antioxidants selenium, choline and carotene. The benefits can be enhanced further by serving it with steamed spinach, grilled tomatoes and mushrooms.

Serves 1   **Preparation time:** 10 minutes   **Cooking time:** 10 minutes

½ avocado
a dash of lemon juice
2 large eggs
1 wholemeal muffin, halved
a little butter, for spreading
freshly ground black pepper

1 Fill a poaching pan 4cm/1½in deep with water and add two poaching rings to the pan. Bring to the boil over a high heat.

2 While it is boiling, peel, pit and slice the avocado and toss with the lemon juice.

3 Turn the heat down to low, break the eggs into the poaching rings, cover and simmer for 3–4 minutes until the whites of the eggs are opaque and firm to touch.

4 Meanwhile, heat the grill/broiler and toast the muffin, then spread the cut sides with butter. Put a poached egg on top of each muffin half, sprinkle with a little pepper and serve hot with the avocado.

Nutrition facts (per serving) Calories 503   Carbohydrate 36g
Protein 21.7g   Fat 30g (of which saturates 7.6g)

Buckwheat Pancakes with Strawberries & Vanilla Yogurt

Using buckwheat for these pancakes makes them a useful wheat-free option, as well as giving the dish the slightly more nutty flavour and texture that I prefer. Buckwheat is also a great source of complex carbohydrate, making these pancakes a perfect choice before a hard training session.

Serves 4 **Preparation time:** 10 minutes, plus 30 minutes' resting (optional)
Cooking time: 15 minutes

270ml/9½fl oz/generous 1 cup skimmed milk
1 egg
a pinch of sea salt
115g/4oz/scant 1 cup buckwheat flour
3 tbsp rapeseed/canola oil
200g/7oz strawberries, hulled and chopped
400g/14oz/1⅔ cups low-fat vanilla yogurt

1 Put the milk, egg and salt in a large bowl and mix together well.

2 Sift the buckwheat flour into a separate bowl. Gradually add the flour to the milk mixture, stirring constantly until you have a smooth batter. You can make the pancakes straight away or cover the batter and leave to rest in the fridge for 30 minutes.

3 Heat a pancake or frying pan until hot, then add 1 teaspoon of the oil and swirl to coat the base of the pan. Pour in about 3 tablespoons of the pancake mixture and again swirl the pan to spread it evenly over the base. Cook for 1–2 minutes until golden underneath, then flip over and brown the other side. Remove from the pan and keep warm. Continue to fry 7 more pancakes, layering the cooked pancakes with baking paper and keeping them warm while you cook.

4 Put a handful of chopped strawberries and 2 heaped tablespoons vanilla yogurt into the centre of each pancake and fold into a triangle to serve.

Nutrition facts (per serving) Calories 314 Carbohydrate 34.5g
Protein 13g Fat 13.9g (of which saturates 2.3g)

Oaty Banana Pancake

Another alternative to the traditional batter pancake, this recipe is relatively fuss-free so is great to make in the morning, even before work. Oats are the main ingredient, they are packed full of slow-release carbohydrate and soluble fibre, ensuring that you not only stay full until lunchtime but you are also less likely to reach for the biscuit barrel or cookie jar mid-afternoon. That also means it gives you plenty of stamina as a pre-training option.

Serves 1 **Preparation time:** 5 minutes **Cooking time:** 8 minutes

100g/3½oz/1 cup rolled oats
1 egg
1 tbsp low-fat soft cheese
2 tbsp skimmed milk
1 banana, chopped
2 tsp clear honey

1 Put the oats, egg, cream cheese and milk in a bowl and whisk until you have a smooth batter.

2 Heat a non-stick frying pan over a medium heat, then pour in half the batter and cook for 4 minutes, or until the pancake is set around the edge with some bubbles through the centre. Flip it over and cook on the other side until golden and set.

3 Serve with chopped banana and a drizzle of honey.

Nutrition facts (per serving) Calories 371 Carbohydrate 57g Protein 17g
Fat 9.2g (of which saturates 1.3g)

LIGHT MEALS

Thai Green Chicken Curry

This is a great dish to come home to after a training session. The chicken provides much-needed protein to help muscles recover and repair, while the spices add essential antioxidants to help prevent further stress on the body. If you are recovering from a high-intensity session, serve the curry with a pitta bread.

Serves 4   **Preparation time:** 10 minutes   **Cooking time:** 25 minutes

1 tbsp oil, for frying

2 garlic cloves, finely chopped

1 bunch of spring onions/scallions, finely chopped

185g/6½oz Thai green curry paste

400g/14oz skinless, boneless chicken breast, diced

400ml/14fl oz/generous 1½ cups coconut milk

100g/3½oz fine green beans

100g/3½oz carrots, cut into batons

200g/7oz spinach leaves

2 large courgettes/zucchini, cut into chunks

juice of ½ lime

1 handful of coriander/cilantro leaves, chopped

1 small red chilli, deseeded and chopped (optional)

1 Heat the oil in a wok or large frying pan over a medium heat, add the garlic and spring onions/scallions and fry for a few minutes until they are golden brown. Add the curry paste and cook for a further 3 minutes, stirring occasionally, or until you can smell their aroma.

2 Add the chicken and stir to coat well with the paste.

3 Add the coconut milk and 400ml/14fl oz/generous 1½ cups water, turn the heat up to high and bring to the boil, then turn the heat down to low and simmer for 10 minutes.

4 Add the remaining vegetables and simmer for 8 minutes, or until the chicken and vegetables are just tender. Add the lime juice, coriander/cilantro and chilli for extra spice, if you like.

5 Serve straight away or leave to cool, put in an airtight container and store in the fridge until needed.

Nutrition facts (per serving) Calories 347 Carbohydrate 15g Protein 20g
Fat 25g (of which saturates 15.7g)

Chicken & Quinoa Salad

This salad is a great choice to take to work if you have an evening training session planned, or to cook after a late workout when you don't want to spend ages preparing a meal. Quinoa is a slow-release carbohydrate; additionally it is one of the only grains with a high protein content. I have suggested the use of walnut oil here, which adds a nutty taste but also provides omega-3 fats, which can be useful in preventing fatigue.

Serves 4   **Preparation time:** 15 minutes, plus 20 minutes cooling
Cooking time: 15 minutes

150g/5½oz/¾ cup quinoa
1 litre/35fl oz/4 cups chicken stock
400g/14oz skinless, boneless, cooked
  chicken, cut into chunks
150g/5½oz cherry tomatoes
100g/3½oz cucumber, chopped

1 red or green pepper, deseeded
  and chopped
1 tbsp walnut oil
1 avocado
juice of ½ lemon
sea salt and freshly ground
  black pepper

1 Put the quinoa and stock in a saucepan and bring to the boil over a high heat, then turn the heat down to low and simmer for 12 minutes, or until the quinoa is soft and has absorbed most of the stock. Drain off any remaining stock, put the quinoa in a bowl and leave to cool.

2 Add the chicken, tomatoes, cucumber, pepper and oil, season with salt and pepper and toss together to mix.

3 Peel the avocado, remove the pit and cut the flesh into chunks. Toss with the lemon juice, then gently fold into the salad. Serve straight away or put in an airtight container and chill in the fridge for up to 3 days.

Nutrition facts (per serving)   Calories 408   Carbohydrate 33.5g
Protein 30.5g   Fat 17.6g (of which saturates 3.9g)

Chicken Kebabs with Spiced Tahini

This healthy option means you don't have to miss out on a barbecue just because you are training for an event. Chicken provides a great source of lean protein, while the tahini sauce not only adds flavour but also provides calcium, which is essential for bone health.

Serves 4   **Preparation time:** 15 minutes   **Cooking time:** 10 minutes

4 skinless, boneless chicken breasts, cut into 5cm/2in cubes

1 red pepper, deseeded and cut into chunks

1 yellow pepper, deseeded and cut into chunks

1 red onion, cut into chunks

250g/9oz mushrooms

1 tbsp olive oil

mixed salad or roasted vegetables, to serve

For the Spiced Tahini:

½ tsp cumin seeds

1 tbsp tahini

juice of ½ lemon

½ tsp paprika

1 To make the Spiced Tahini, put the cumin seeds in a dry saucepan over a medium heat and toss for a few minutes until just beginning to brown. Leave to cool slightly, then mix with all the remaining tahini ingredients.

2 Preheat the barbecue or grill/broiler.

3 Thread the chicken, peppers, onion and mushrooms alternately onto eight kebab skewers. Brush lightly with oil. Barbecue or grill/broil for about 10 minutes, turning regularly, until browned on the outside and the chicken is cooked through.

4 Serve with the spiced tahini and a mixed salad or roasted vegetables.

Nutrition facts (per serving) Calories 251 Carbohydrate 10g Protein 32g Fat 9g (of which saturates 1.6g)

Beef Soba Noodles

Red meat is a great source of dietary iron but we often miss out on this valuable nutrient because we are wary of too much saturated fat. The solution is to choose a lean fillet of beef. Bottles of sweet chilli sauce are available in the supermarket.

Serves 4 **Preparation time:** 15 minutes **Cooking time:** 15 minutes

200g/7oz soba noodles

2 tbsp rapeseed/canola oil

400g/14oz beef fillet, thinly sliced

3 spring onions/scallions, sliced
  into rings

1 small red pepper, deseeded and sliced

1 carrot, sliced lengthways into batons

100g/7oz mangetout/snow peas,
  halved lengthways

200g/7oz baby corn, halved lengthways

125ml/4fl oz/½ cup sweet chilli sauce

2 tbsp soy sauce

2 tbsp lime juice

1 Put the noodles in a large, heatproof bowl and cover with boiling water. Leave to stand for 2 minutes, using a wooden spoon to gently separate strands. Drain well and leave to one side.

2 Heat the oil in a wok or large frying pan over a high heat. Add the beef a few pieces at a time and stir-fry for a few minutes until browned and tender, then set aside while you brown the remaining beef.

3 Add the spring onions/scallions to the wok with 1 tablespoon water and stir-fry for 2 minutes, or until tender. Add all the other vegetables and continue to stir-fry for 4 minutes, or until just soft but still with a slight crunch. Stir in the noodles.

4 Mix together the chilli sauce, soy sauce and lime juice, then add it to the wok and toss to coat all the ingredients. Cook for a further 3 minutes, or until heated through. Return the beef to the wok and stir-fry for 2–3 minutes until hot. Serve straight away.

Nutrition facts (per serving) Calories 477 Carbohydrate 59g
Protein 31.5g Fat 14.8g (of which saturates 10g)

Spicy Steak Wraps with Tomato Salsa

Wraps make a great alternative to sandwiches and this one is also a good way to use up leftovers. Although red meat has had a bad press recently, it is still the best source of iron available so should be included in your diet in moderation. By choosing a lean steak, you will take on a great source of protein with minimal saturated fat. The salsa is packed full of lycopene-rich tomatoes and red peppers, not forgetting chilli, which is a potent source of capsaicin, known for its antioxidant and anti-inflammatory properties. Further research also suggests a potential role for capsinoids in weight maintenance and improved body fat composition. Plus there's some evidence that chilli can help eliminate congestion, boost immunity and prevent stomach ulcers.

Serves 2   Preparation time: 10 minutes

2 lean beef steaks, each 150g/5½oz
1 red pepper, deseeded and sliced
2 wholemeal tortilla wraps

For the Tomato Salsa:
1 small onion
1 red chilli, deseeded

1 garlic clove
1 beef/beefsteak tomato, chopped
2 tsp balsamic vinegar
1 handful of coriander/cilantro leaves, chopped

1 Preheat the grill/broiler. Grill/broil the steaks for 2–3 minutes on each side, depending on the thickness of the steaks, until they are cooked to your preferred doneness.

2 To make the salsa, put the onion, chilli and garlic in a food processor and whiz until finely chopped, almost paste-like. Add the tomato, vinegar and coriander/cilantro and mix together well.

3 Place a steak in the centre of each wrap and divide the sliced peppers and salsa equally between the wraps. Fold the tortillas to encase the filling. Serve straight away, or wrap in cling film/plastic wrap and serve as a portable meal.

Nutrition facts (per serving)   Calories 403   Carbohydrate 37g
Protein 37.5g   Fat 10g (of which saturates 4.4g)

Salmon Muscle-Recovery Wraps

Once training is over, it is essential to think about muscle recovery. Studies show the optimal time for this is within 2 hours of finishing training, but the earlier the better. It is well documented that omega-3 fats help to reduce inflammation but they can also be beneficial in reducing fatigue, so why not try this wrap specially designed for the purpose? The wholemeal tortilla will help to replenish glycogen stores, while the avocado provides further essential fats, the tomatoes include lycopene and there's vitamin B6 from the lettuce.

Serves 2   **Preparation time:** 10 minutes

200g/7oz grilled or canned salmon, skinned and flaked
2 tbsp plain yogurt
1½ tbsp lime juice
2 wholemeal tortilla wraps
½ avocado, peeled, pitted and sliced
2 large tomatoes, sliced
2 handfuls of shredded lettuce

1 Mix the salmon with the yogurt and lime juice.

2 Divide the salmon mixture equally between the wraps and top each one with half the avocado, tomato and lettuce. Roll and fold each wrap to encase the filling. Serve straight away, or wrap in cling film/plastic wrap for a portable meal.

Nutrition facts (per serving) Calories 534 Carbohydrate 51.8g
Protein 32.5g Fat 23.1g (of which saturates 4.6g)

Salmon Chowder

This hearty, all-in-one meal is one of my favourite ways to recover from a training session on a cold morning. The salmon provides protein and omega-3 fats for tired muscles, while the potatoes start to replace depleted glycogen stores.

Serves 4 **Preparation time:** 15 minutes **Cooking time:** 30 minutes

1 tbsp rapeseed/canola oil
1 large onion, roughly chopped
1 large floury potato, such as Maris
   Piper, peeled and finely diced
1 fennel bulb
500ml/17fl oz/2 cups fish or
   vegetable stock
250ml/9fl oz/1 cup skimmed milk

300g/10½oz salmon fillet, skinned
   and cut into 5cm/2in pieces
100g/3½oz/generous ⅓ cup
   plain yogurt
1 small bunch of chives,
   roughly chopped
sea salt and freshly ground
   black pepper

1 Heat the oil in a saucepan over a medium heat, add the onion and fry for about 3 minutes until softened but not browned. Add the potato and cook for a further 3 minutes.

2 Cut the feathery tops off the fennel and keep for later. Cut the rest of the fennel in half, remove the core, then finely chop the bulb. Add the chopped fennel and stock to the pan and season with salt and pepper. Bring to the boil, then turn the heat down to low, cover and simmer for 5–8 minutes until the potato is tender.

3 Gently stir in the milk and salmon pieces and simmer for a further 10 minutes, or until the salmon flakes easily when tested with a fork. Add the yogurt, fennel tops and chives and simmer for a further 10 minutes, uncovered, until the chowder is thick and well blended.

4 Ladle the chowder into bowls and serve hot, or leave to cool and reheat gently when you are ready to serve.

Nutrition facts (per serving) Calories 286 Carbohydrate 26.8
Protein 22.8g Fat 10.1g (of which saturates 1.7g)

Smoked Haddock
& Squash Fishcakes

Haddock is not only high in lean protein, magnesium, vitamins B6, B12 and niacin, it's also reasonably priced and very tasty. This recipe is one the whole family will enjoy and is a great way to introduce fish to children. By using butternut squash instead of the usual potato, the carbohydrate content is reduced, making these fishcakes ideal for a low-intensity or rest day. The squash can be replaced with sweet potato if you want to use this recipe on a moderate or high-intensity day. Serve the fishcakes just as they are, or with wholemeal pitta bread and a colourful side salad.

Serves 4　**Preparation time:** 15 minutes, plus 30 minutes' chilling
Cooking time: 20 minutes

300g/11oz butternut squash, peeled, deseeded and cut into chunks
250g/9oz hot-smoked haddock fillets
1 tsp chopped chilli
4 spring onions/scallions, chopped (optional)
2 tbsp defrosted, frozen peas or sweetcorn/corn kernels (optional)

1 tbsp chopped coriander/cilantro leaves (optional)
wholemeal bread flour, for dusting
1 tbsp rapeseed/canola oil, for frying
sea salt and freshly ground black pepper
chopped cucumber, cherry tomatoes and chopped pepper, to serve

1　Put the butternut squash in a saucepan and cover with water. Bring to the boil over a high heat, then turn the heat down to low and simmer for 10 minutes, or until soft. Drain well, then mash. You should have about 250g/9oz mashed squash.

2　Flake the haddock and mix with the mashed squash. Season with salt and pepper, add your choice of the optional ingredients and mix together well. Shape into eight patties and chill in the fridge for at least 30 minutes.

3　Dust the patties with the flour, shaking off any excess. Heat the oil in a frying pan over a medium heat and fry for 5 minutes, or until golden brown on both sides. Drain on paper towels and serve hot or cold with chopped cucumber, cherry tomatoes and peppers.

Nutrition facts (per serving)　Calories 156　Carbohydrate 20g
Protein 18.5g　Fat 6g (of which saturates 0.8g)

Prawn & Orange Salad

Oranges are high in vitamin C and they make a perfect accompaniment to prawns/shrimp. These shellfish are an excellent source of protein and potent antioxidants, vitamin E and selenium, making this salad an excellent light recovery meal.

Serves 4   **Preparation time:** 10 minutes

150g/5½oz mixed salad leaves

3 oranges, divided into segments

1 ripe avocado, peeled, pitted and cut into chunks

250g/9oz cooked king prawns/ jumbo shrimp

1 red onion, finely chopped

1 raw beetroot/beet, peeled and grated

50g/2oz/½ cup walnuts, chopped

For the Walnut Dressing:

1 tbsp walnut oil

1 tsp clear honey

juice of ½ lime

a pinch of herbes de Provence

1 Put all the salad ingredients in a large salad bowl and toss them together lightly.

2 Whisk together the dressing ingredients in a small jug, or put them in a screw-topped jar, seal and shake well to combine. Drizzle over the salad, toss and serve straight away.

3 Alternatively, if you are not serving the salad straight away, keep the dressing separate until you are ready to eat.

Nutrition facts (per serving) Calories 240 Carbohydrate 24.1g Protein 17.9g Fat 9.4g (of which saturates 0.8g)

Tortilla Pizzas

This pizza is not only nutrient packed, the addition of the sweet potato makes it a great pre-exercise meal as it is high in slow-release carbohydrate, which will give you sustained energy and keep your blood-sugar levels constant. Keep the skin on the sweet potatoes for maximum nutrient retention.

Serves 4   **Preparation time:** 10 minutes   **Cooking time:** 20 minutes

2 sweet potatoes (about 600g/1lb 5oz total weight),
    cut into 2.5cm/1in cubes
1 tbsp olive oil
1 mild red chilli, deseeded and chopped
4 large wholemeal tortillas
6 spring onions/scallions, sliced
200g/7oz/1⅓ cups feta cheese, crumbled
sea salt and freshly ground black pepper
mixed green salad, to serve

1 Preheat the oven to 200°C/400°F/Gas 6.

2 Put the sweet potatoes in a roasting pan, pour over the oil, sprinkle with the chilli and toss together to coat the sweet potato chunks. Roast for 15–20 minutes until browned and tender.

3 Reduce the oven temp to 180°C/350°F/Gas 4 and put the tortillas on two large baking sheets. Spoon the sweet potato over the tortillas, then scatter with the spring onions/scallions and the feta cheese. Season with salt and pepper. Return the pizzas to the oven for 8–10 minutes until the cheese has melted and they begin to turn golden.

4 Serve with a green salad.

Nutrition facts (per serving) Calories 545 Carbohydrate 79g
Protein 16.8g Fat 18.1g (of which saturates 9.6g)

Courgette & Feta Frittata

I love this recipe as it is so simple and can actually be done with any combination of vegetables and herbs that you might have in the fridge, garden or pantry. Eggs are one of my favourite foods as they are a powerhouse of nutrients. Two large eggs provide you with your daily 20g protein, plus they are recommended for recovery because they have a high-satiety factor, which means they help keep you full and prevent you from getting the munchies!

Serves 4   **Preparation time:** 10 minutes   **Cooking time:** 8 minutes

6 eggs

1 tbsp skimmed milk

a pinch of dried oregano

1 tbsp rapeseed/canola oil

1 cm/½in piece of root ginger, peeled and finely chopped

1–2 garlic cloves, finely chopped

2 courgettes/zucchini, sliced

100g/3½oz/⅔ cup feta cheese, crumbled

sea salt and freshly ground black pepper

mixed green salad, to serve

1 Whisk together the eggs and milk in a large bowl and season with oregano, salt and pepper, then leave to one side.

2 Heat the oil in a large frying pan over a low heat. Add the ginger and garlic and fry for about 3 minutes until golden brown, stirring regularly. Add the courgettes/zucchini and cook for a further 3–5 minutes until they are also golden in colour.

3 Preheat the grill/broiler to medium-high.

4 Pour the egg mixture into the pan and cook over a medium heat for a few minutes until it looks like it will come away from the sides of the pan. Scatter over the feta. Remove the pan from the heat and put under the hot grill/broiler for 3 minutes, or until the top is golden. Cut into quarters and serve hot with a mixed green salad.

Nutrition facts (per serving)   Calories 240   Carbohydrate 5.2g   Protein 16g Fat 17.8g (of which saturates 6.8g)

Egg Fried Rice with Toasted Cashews

Another great quick and easy-to-prepare recovery meal, you'll love this after a high-intensity training session. It is even quicker if you some leftover cooked long-grain rice, in which case you can start at step 2.

Serves 4   **Preparation time:** 10 minutes   **Cooking time:** 25 minutes

200g/7oz/scant 1 cup brown rice

100g/3½oz/scant 1 cup cashew nuts

1 tbsp rapeseed/canola oil

2 garlic cloves, finely chopped

1 large carrot, thinly sliced

100g/3½oz/¾ cup frozen sweetcorn/
   corn kernels

100g/3½oz/¾ cup frozen peas

3 eggs, lightly beaten

2 tsp soy sauce

1 tbsp chopped coriander/
   cilantro leaves

freshly ground black pepper

1 Put the rice in a saucepan and cover with cold water. Bring to the boil over a high heat, then partially cover, turn the heat down to low and simmer for 14 minutes, or until the rice is just tender but still has a little bite. Drain and rinse in cold water, then leave in a colander to drain and cool.

2 Meanwhile, put the cashews in a dry frying pan over a medium heat and toss for a few minutes until just beginning to brown. Tip out and leave to one side.

3 Heat the oil in a large frying pan over a medium heat, add the garlic and fry for 3 minutes, stirring gently, or until golden in colour. Add the carrot, sweetcorn/corn and peas and cook for 2–3 minutes, stirring occasionally, until well mixed. Stir in the cooked rice.

4 Turn the heat down to low and slowly stir in the eggs so that they mix with the rice and vegetables and cook through. Add the soy sauce, season with pepper to taste, sprinkle with most of the toasted nuts and coriander and stir them into the rice. Spoon into individual serving bowls, sprinkle with the remaining nuts and coriander/cilantro and serve hot.

Nutrition facts (per serving) Calories 460 Carbohydrate 56.5g
Protein 14.4g Fat 20.4g (of which saturates 3.4g)

Hearty Vegetable Soup

This makes a wonderfully warming and filling meal, whether you serve it on its own at lunch time or before an evening training session, or combine it with some fresh sourdough or rye bread after training to make it into a main recovery meal.

Serves 4   **Preparation time:** 10 minutes   **Cooking time:** 25 minutes

1 tbsp rapeseed/canola oil

1 onion, chopped

2 garlic cloves, chopped

2 carrots, chopped

4 celery stalks, chopped

½ butternut squash (about 300g/10½oz prepared weight), peeled, deseeded and chopped

1 litre/35fl oz/4 cups vegetable stock

400g/14oz canned chopped tomatoes

1 tsp dried oregano

1 tsp paprika

400g/14oz canned butter/lima beans, drained and rinsed

2 tbsp chopped parsley leaves

1 Heat the oil in a large saucepan over a medium heat and fry the onion for 3 minutes, or until soft. Add the garlic and cook for 1 minute. Add the carrot, celery and butternut squash and stir into the onion mixture.

2 Add the stock, tomatoes and oregano, and bring to the boil. Turn the heat down to low and simmer, partially covered, for 15–20 minutes until the vegetables are tender.

3 Stir in the butter/lima beans and heat through for a few minutes. Stir in the parsley and serve hot.

Nutrition facts (per serving) Calories 201 Carbohydrate 33g Protein 7.5g Fat 4.5g (of which saturates 0.7g)

Chickpea & Kale Broth

Kale is a nutrient-dense vegetable, high in vitamins A and K and – most importantly for sportspeople – a great source of nitrate. The body turns nitrate into nitric oxide, which has been linked to an increased uptake of oxygen into the muscles. Combined with chickpeas and sweet potato, which both help release energy at a slower rate, this dish is tailor-made for pre-training.

Serves 4   **Preparation time:** 10 minutes   **Cooking time:** 1 hour

1 tbsp rapeseed/canola oil

1 tsp cumin seeds

1 large onion, chopped

2 garlic cloves, crushed

1cm/½in piece of root ginger, peeled and finely chopped

1 large sweet potato (about 300g/10½oz), chopped

1 red chilli, deseeded and chopped (optional)

1 litre/35fl oz/4 cups vegetable stock

1 large bunch of curly kale, washed and torn into smaller pieces

800g/1lb 12oz canned chickpeas, drained and rinsed

1 Heat the oil in a large saucepan over a medium heat. Add the cumin seeds and shake the pan for a minute or so until you can smell their aroma. Add the onion, garlic and ginger and fry for 4–5 minutes, stirring occasionally, until golden brown.

2 Add the sweet potato and chilli, if using, and cook for a further 5 minutes.

3 Pour in the stock and bring to the boil, then turn the heat down to low and simmer for 15–20 minutes until the sweet potato is tender.

4 Add the kale and simmer for a further 20 minutes. Add the chickpeas and simmer for 5 more minutes, stirring occasionally, or until everything is heated through and well blended. Serve hot.

Nutrition facts (per serving) Calories 294 Carbohydrate 47.9g
Protein 14.4g Fat 5.9g (of which saturates 0.5g)

Sweet Potato & Red Lentil Soup

I love this soup and it tends to be a staple in our house during the winter months. Packed full of slow-release carbohydrate and iron-rich lentils, it is the perfect lunch choice after a really tough morning training session out in the cold and wet.

Serves 4   **Preparation time:** 10 minutes   **Cooking time:** 35 minutes

1 tbsp rapeseed/canola oil

1 red onion, chopped

1 garlic clove, crushed

4 sweet potatoes (about 1.2kg/2lb 12oz
   total weight) peeled and chopped

85g/3oz/⅓ cup red lentils

1 litre/35fl oz/4 cups vegetable stock

½ tsp paprika

½ tsp ground cumin

½ tsp chilli powder

1 handful of coriander/cilantro
   leaves, chopped

1 Heat the oil in a large saucepan over a medium heat. Add the onion and garlic and cook for 2–3 minutes until tender. Add the sweet potatoes and red lentils and cook for 2 minutes.

2 Add the stock, paprika, cumin and chilli powder, bring to the boil, then turn the heat down to low and simmer for 30 minutes, or until the sweet potatoes are tender and the lentils are cooked.

3 Blend using a hand-held blender or transfer to a blender or food processor and whiz until smooth. Sprinkle with the coriander/cilantro and serve hot.

Nutrition facts (per serving) Calories 384 Carbohydrate 76g
Protein 12.2g Fat 3.9g (of which saturates 0.6g)

Three-Lentil Dhal with Coriander & Chilli

This recipe is inspired by my mum. She is a fantastic cook and makes the best dhal I have ever tasted! I have added a slight twist to her traditional Punjabi recipe with the addition of some coconut milk and by cooking all the spices together at the start. Lentils are often overlooked but they are cheap, very easy to cook and extremely high in soluble fibre, making them a great choice if you are trying to cut calories as they keep you full for ages.

Serves 4   **Preparation time:** 10 minutes   **Cooking time:** 50 minutes

1 tbsp rapeseed/canola oil

1 tsp cumin seeds

2 garlic cloves, crushed

7cm/2¾in piece of root ginger, peeled and finely chopped

1 red chilli, deseeded and chopped

400g/14oz canned chopped tomatoes

1 tsp sea salt

85g/3oz/⅓ cup red lentils

85g/3oz/⅓ cup yellow lentils

85g/3oz/scant ½ cup green lentils

1 handful of coriander/cilantro eaves, chopped

2 tbsp coconut cream

1 Heat the oil in a large saucepan over a medium heat. Add the cumin seeds and shake the pan for a minute or so until you can smell their aroma. Add the garlic, ginger and chilli and fry for about 5 minutes, stirring occasionally, until golden brown.

2 Add the tomatoes and salt, stir well and cook for a further 3 minutes. Stir in all the lentils so they are coated in the tomato mixture, then add 750ml/26fl oz/3 cups boiling water. Turn the heat down to low and simmer for 30–40 minutes until the lentils have soaked up the water and are tender.

3 Sprinkle with coriander/cilantro, top with a dollop of coconut cream and serve hot.

Nutrition facts (per serving) Calories 313 Carbohydrate 38g
Protein 13.6g Fat 12g (of which saturates 3g)

Super Beans on Toast

This was an experimental dish I first made a while back when the cupboards were bare but I needed to put together a quick, light dinner after travelling all day! The yeast extract is optional and can be substituted with soy sauce or even balsamic vinegar if you're not a fan.

Serves 2   **Preparation time:** 5 minutes   **Cooking time:** 5 minutes

400g/14oz canned baked beans
400g/14oz canned kidney beans, drained and rinsed
1 tsp yeast extract (optional)
4 slices of wholemeal or rye bread toast
butter or margarine, for spreading
mixed salad, to serve

1 Heat the baked beans in a saucepan over a medium heat. Stir in the kidney beans and yeast extract until combined and warmed through.

2 Toast the bread, then spread with butter or margarine.

3 Divide the toast between two serving plates, pour over the bean mixture and serve with a mixed salad.

Nutrition facts (per serving) Calories 410 Carbohydrate 59g Protein 18g Fat 11g (of which saturates 5g)

Avocado & Seeded Toasts

I love this combination of avocado and seeds any time of day – I've even been known to have it as a mid-afternoon snack to satisfy the munchies!

Serves 2   **Preparation time:** 5 minutes   **Cooking time:** 5 minutes

1½ tbsp sunflower seeds
4 slices of wholemeal, rye or sourdough bread
1 large avocado, peeled, pitted and roughly chopped
2 tbsp fat-free Greek yogurt
1 large beef/beefsteak tomato, sliced
sea salt and freshly ground black pepper

1 Put the sunflower seeds in a dry frying pan over a medium heat and toast for a few minutes until lightly browned, shaking the pan occasionally. Tip into a bowl.

2 Toast the bread.

3 Add the avocado and yogurt to the bowl and mash together until smooth, then spread over the toast slices. Arrange the slices of tomato over the top of the toasts, sprinkle with the toasted seeds, season, and serve.

Nutrition facts (per serving) Calories 418 Carbohydrate 46g Protein 13g Fat 21.8g (of which saturates 4.5g)

HERO FOOD: AVOCADO

Avocados are probably one of the most under-rated fruits, feared by many due to their high fat and energy content. However, the reality is that they are packed full of those very helpful good fats essential for absorbing fat-soluble vitamins such as vitamins A, D, E and K, and are also a great source of vitamin E itself. So, while a 100g/3½oz serving of avocado provides 160 calories and 15g of fat, only 2g of fat is saturated. The fat content makes it a satisfying choice for those watching their weight. Try it as a snack drizzled with balsamic vinegar, or mashed with some lime, chilli/hot pepper flakes and coriander/cilantro as a topping for toast.

Beetroot & Butternut Panzanella

Colourful and full of flavour, this dish makes a great centrepiece for lunch if you have friends coming over or just fancy a change from a sandwich. It also works towards fuelling your body for a training session later in the day. Beetroot/beet has been widely studied in recent years in the world of sports nutrition. It has a high nitrate content and although the actual concentration varies from beetroot to beetroot and you may not hit the magic 5mmol of nitrate (see page 218), I still like to include it as much as possible before a hard training session.

Serves 4 **Preparation time:** 15 minutes, plus cooling
Cooking time: 30 minutes

500g/1lb 2oz raw beetroot/beets, peeled and cut into chunks

½ butternut squash, peeled, deseeded and cut into chunks

2 tsp dried herbes de Provence

2 tbsp olive oil

6 slices of sourdough bread, roughly torn into chunks

2 garlic cloves, finely chopped

50g/2oz baby spinach leaves

3 tbsp balsamic vinegar

1 Preheat the oven to 200°C/400°F/Gas 6.

2 Put the beetroot/beets, squash, herbs and half the oil in a large bowl and toss together to coat the vegetables in the oil. Spread the mixture on a baking sheet and roast for 25 minutes, or until the vegetables are tender. 3 Meanwhile, tip the bread chunks, garlic and remaining oil into the same bowl and toss well to coat.

4 Once the vegetables are cooked, scatter the bread chunks over the top and roast for a further few minutes until the bread is crisp and golden.

5 Tip the vegetables and bread into a large salad bowl and leave to cool.

6 Just before serving, add the spinach, sprinkle with the balsamic vinegar and toss all the ingredients together.

Nutrition facts (per serving) Calories 287 Carbohydrate 48.3g
Protein 8.5g Fat 8.2g (of which saturates 1.3g)

Mushroom, Spinach & Halloumi Salad

Meeting your daily dairy and calcium requirements as a physically active individual is very important. Studies have shown that those who consumed a higher intake of calcium from dairy products tended to lay down more lean muscle mass than those who did not. That said, some dairy options – like cheese – also have a high saturated fat content so should not be eaten daily and you should focus on those varieties that are naturally lower in fat, such as halloumi, feta and mozzarella. This salad makes a great recovery option from a low-intensity training session or as a choice on a rest day.

Serves 4 **Preparation time:** 10 minutes **Cooking time:** 10 minutes

1 tbsp olive oil

300g/10½oz mushrooms, thickly sliced

1 garlic clove, crushed

300g/10½oz halloumi, drained
  and sliced

150g/5½oz/1 cup cherry tomatoes

150g/5½oz baby spinach leaves

1 handful of basil leaves

1 tbsp balsamic vinegar

1 tsp clear honey

2 tsp dried oregano

1 Heat the oil in a non-stick frying or griddle pan over a medium heat. Add the mushrooms and garlic and fry for a few minutes until the mushrooms soften. Remove from the pan and leave to one side.

2 Add the halloumi slices to the pan and cook for about 4 minutes, turning once, until golden on both sides. Remove from the pan and leave to one side.

3 Put the tomatoes, spinach and basil in a large salad bowl. Add the mushrooms and halloumi and toss gently to combine.

4 Mix together the balsamic vinegar, honey and oregano in a small jug, then pour over salad and serve straight away.

Nutrition facts (per serving) Calories 311 Carbohydrate 10g Protein 20g Fat 22.8g (of which saturates 13.9g)

Beetroot, Feta & Potato Salad

A great light supper after training, with a good dairy source of protein.

Serves 4   **Preparation time:** 15 minutes   **Cooking time:** 1 hour

2 baking potatoes, scrubbed

100g/3½oz mini pickled beetroot/beets, drained

150g/5½oz mixed salad leaves

200g/7oz/1⅔ cups cubed feta cheese

50g/1¾oz cucumber, cubed

150g/5½oz/1 cup cherry tomatoes

1 large carrot, sliced

85g/3oz/scant 1 cup green olives with chilli (optional)

1 handful of coriander/cilantro leaves, chopped

balsamic vinegar, to serve

walnut oil, to serve

1 Preheat the oven to 200°C/400°F/Gas 6. Pierce the potatoes with a fork, then bake for 1 hour, or until soft on the inside with a lovely crisp skin. Meanwhile combine all the other salad ingredients in a large salad bowl.

2 Remove the potatoes from the oven. Leave to cool for 10 minutes, then cut into chunks and add to the salad. Toss all the ingredients together. Serve with the vinegar and oil on the side so everyone can add their own.

Nutrition facts (per serving without dressing) Calories 286
Carbohydrate 35g   Protein 11.2g   Fat 12.4g (of which saturates 7.7g)

HERO FOOD: BEETROOT/ BEETS

In recent years, there has been much hype about the use of beetroot as a performance aid. Studies have demonstrated that the high nitrate content of beetroot encourages oxygen uptake by up to 16 per cent, thus preventing the build-up of acidity and improving performance at high intensities. Studies conclude that a daily consumption of 5mmol of nitrate 1–3 hours before training, prior to competing in events lasting 3–36 minutes are required for this desired performance effect. One main issue is that the nitrate content within beetroot differs, making it difficult to determine how much to eat to meet this 5mmol requirement. Specific beetroot shots/juices have been developed with this in mind, but they are an acquired taste!

Roasted Vegetable & Mozzarella Bruschetta

This is a Mediterranean twist on the humble cheese on toast. It's easy and quick, plus it provides you with the benefits of vegetables rich in antioxidants. Sourdough makes exceptionally good and crisp toast and adds to the overall flavour of this light meal.

Serves 4   **Preparation time:** 5 minutes   **Cooking time:** 15 minutes

2 courgettes/zucchini, sliced
2 red peppers, deseeded and
  cut into chunks
1 aubergine/eggplant, sliced
100g/3½oz mushrooms, sliced
4 garlic cloves, finely chopped

1 tbsp dried oregano
3 tbsp rapeseed/canola oil
8 slices of sourdough bread
200g/7oz mozzarella cheese, sliced
freshly ground black pepper

1 Preheat the grill/broiler to medium.

2 Put all the vegetables and the garlic on a grill tray, sprinkle with the oregano and drizzle the oil over the top. Toss together so all the vegetables are lightly coated. Grill/broil for 8–10 minutes, turning the vegetables occasionally, until they are soft and golden.

3 Toast the bread.

4 Spoon the vegetables onto the slices of toast and cover with slices of mozzarella. Put back under the grill/broiler for 5 minutes, or until the cheese has melted. Season with black pepper and serve hot.

Nutrition facts (per serving) Calories 459   Carbohydrate 45.7g
Protein 24.5g   Fat 21.1g (of which saturates 6.5g)

Roast Sweet Potato & Spinach Wraps with Tomato Salsa

A great light option, this also makes an ideal portable meal for when you are travelling to an event later in the day. The sweet potato and wholemeal tortilla will provide you with plenty of slow-release carbohydrate to fuel your high-intensity session, competition or just straight training. Of course, if you already have some cooked sweet potatoes, the recipe is even quicker and easier.

Serves 2　Preparation time: 10 minutes　Cooking time: 1 hour

1 sweet potato, about 250g/9oz, cut into chunks
1 handful of baby spinach leaves
2 wholemeal tortilla wraps
Tomato Salsa (see page 202)
freshly ground black pepper

1　Preheat the oven to 200°C/400°F/Gas 6.

2　Pierce the potato several times with a fork, then bake for 1 hour, or until soft on the inside with a lovely crisp skin. Leave to cool, then cut into chunks.

3　Divide the sweet potato chunks and spinach between the wraps. Add 1 tablespoon Tomato Salsa to each wrap and season with black pepper. Roll up or fold the wraps and eat straight away or wrap in cling film/plastic wrap and keep in the fridge until later.

Nutrition facts (per serving)　Calories 308　Carbohydrate 60g　Protein 8.5g
Fat 3.2g (of which saturates 1.2g)

Root Vegetable Chips with Dippy Eggs

This is a real favourite and it demonstrates how training food can include the whole family. It is also what I call a very low-maintenance meal as it is all cooked in one baking pan – which means less washing up, too! If you are serving this as a recovery meal, then make sure you have two eggs to get your 20g of recovery protein.

Serves 4   **Preparation time:** 10 minutes   **Cooking time:** 45 minutes

1 large floury potato, such as Maris Piper, cut into long strips

1 large sweet potato, cut into long strips

2 parsnips, peeled and cut into long strips

2 large carrots, cut into long strips

2 tbsp rapeseed/canola oil

2 tsp dried rosemary

2 tsp clear honey

4 eggs

1 Preheat the oven to 180°C/350°F/Gas 4.

2 Put all the vegetables in a large baking pan. Mix together the oil, rosemary and honey, then pour the mixture over the vegetables and stir well to coat.

3 Cook for about 40 minutes until the vegetables are almost tender.

4 Remove the baking pan from the oven and make 4 spaces among the vegetables. Crack an egg into each space and return the pan to the oven for about 2–3 minutes until the whites of the eggs have turned opaque but the yolks are still runny. Serve straight away.

Nutrition facts (per serving) Calories 215   Carbohydrate 30g   Protein 8.3g
Fat 11.6g (of which saturates 1.6g)

MAIN MEALS

One-Pot Chicken Casserole

When you are juggling training with a job and perhaps a family, main meals must not only meet your training requirements but also suit your lifestyle. This is a great recipe as the complete meal is made in one pot – plus you can even prepare it the night before and have it ready in the fridge to pop into the oven when you get in from work or training. It's also a good one for your slow cooker, if you have one. An ideal recovery choice, it is full of lean protein and carbohydrate to replace glycogen stores.

Serves 4   **Preparation time:** 15 minutes   **Cooking time:** 1 hour

4 skinless, boneless chicken breasts

1 large onion, cut into chunks 4 large carrots, cut into chunks

2 large parsnips, peeled and cut into chunks

2 baking potatoes, such as Maris Piper, peeled and cut into chunks

2 garlic cloves, crushed

juice of 1 orange

1 tbsp clear honey

1 handful of rosemary leaves

1 litre/35fl oz/4 cups chicken stock

sea salt and freshly ground black pepper

1 Preheat the oven to 180°C/350°F/Gas 4.

2 Put the chicken breasts into a large casserole dish and surround with the onion, carrots, parsnips and potatoes. Mix together the garlic, orange juice, honey and rosemary and stir into the dish. Finally, pour the stock over the chicken and vegetables and season with salt and pepper.

3 Cover and cook for 45–60 minutes until the vegetables are all cooked through and the chicken juices run clear when pierced with a sharp knife. Serve hot.

Nutrition facts (per serving) Calories 386 Carbohydrate 54.8g
Protein 32.4g Fat 5.3g (of which saturates 1.9g)

Mustard-Mash Chicken Pie

I associate mashed potato with comfort food but it can be a training food with a few adjustments. By replacing the usual high-fat butter and cheese with cream cheese and mustard, you get a lower-fat alternative that's equally flavoursome. The potato skin is nutritious and adds a delicious crunch. Serve this easy one-pot meal to family or friends and they'd never know that you were following a specific nutrition plan.

Serves 4   Preparation time: 15 minutes   **Cooking time:** 1¼ hours

1 tbsp rapeseed/canola oil

4 skinless, boneless chicken breasts, cut into chunks

1 onion, chopped

2 carrots, diced

2 courgettes/zucchini, diced

100g/3½oz runner beans, cut into strips

100g/3½oz/¾ cup fresh, podded, or frozen peas

455ml/16fl oz/scant 2 cups chicken stock

sea salt and freshly ground black pepper

For the Mustard Mash:

750g/1lb 10oz floury potatoes, such as Maris Piper, unpeeled, cut into chunks

30g/1oz low-fat cream cheese

1 tsp wholegrain mustard

2–4 tbsp skimmed milk

1 Preheat the oven to 180°C/350°F/Gas 4.

2 Heat the oil in a frying pan over a low heat, add the chicken and onion and fry for about 5 minutes, stirring occasionally, until brown on all sides.

3 Use a slotted spoon to transfer the chicken and onion to a casserole dish. Add the other vegetables, stock, salt and pepper. Cover and bake for 35–40 minutes until the vegetables are tender and the sauce has thickened.

4 Meanwhile, prepare the mash. Put the potatoes in a large saucepan and cover with water. Cover and bring to the boil over a high heat, then turn the heat down to low and simmer for 10 minutes, or until tender. Drain well, then return to the pan. Add the cream cheese, mustard and enough milk to mash to a smooth mash.

5 Remove the casserole lid and pile the mash on top of the chicken and vegetables, then return the dish to the oven for a further 15–20 minutes until the topping is browned and crisp. Serve hot.

Nutrition facts (per serving) Calories 408 Carbohydrate 44g Protein 34g
Fat 10.9g (of which saturates 4.1g)

Chicken & Cannellini Stroganoff

Beans and pulses are highly nutritious so we shouldn't make the common mistake of overlooking them. They provide both protein and slow-release carbohydrate, as well as being very reasonably priced. Adding the cannellini beans means that you can use less rice while still meeting your carbohydrate requirements.

Serves 4   **Preparation time:** 15 minutes, plus 20 minutes' soaking
Cooking time: 40 minutes

30g/1oz dried porcini mushrooms
1 tbsp rapeseed/canola oil
1 large onion, chopped
1–2 garlic cloves, chopped
3 celery stalks, chopped
300g/10½oz skinless, boneless chicken breasts, cut into chunks
150ml/5fl oz/scant ⅔ cup chicken or vegetable stock

2 tsp wholegrain mustard
¼ tsp paprika
200g/7oz canned cannellini beans, drained and rinsed
sea salt and freshly ground black pepper
100g/3½oz/heaped ½ cup brown rice, to serve

1 Put the mushrooms in a bowl, cover with 200ml/7fl oz/¾ cup boiling water and leave to soak for 20 minutes.

2 Heat the oil in a large, non-stick saucepan over a medium heat. Add the onion, garlic, celery and chicken and fry for 2–3 minutes, stirring regularly, until just browned.

3 Add the soaked mushrooms with their soaking liquid, the stock, mustard, paprika and beans, then season with salt and pepper. Cover, bring to the boil over a high heat, then turn down the heat to low and simmer for 30 minutes until the chicken is cooked through and the juice has reduced to a thick sauce.

4 Meanwhile, cook the rice in boiling water for about 30 minutes until just tender, then drain and serve with the stroganoff.

Nutrition facts (per serving) Calories 477 Carbohydrate 56.8g
Protein 37.7g Fat 10.2g (of which saturates 2.4g)

Tangy Chicken Stir-Fry

A stir-fry is one of the easiest, most versatile and nutritious ways of cooking food. Choose your protein – whether it's tofu, beans, fish or chicken – pick a variety of vegetables, herbs and spices and away you go. Serve with noodles or rice for a well-balanced training meal any evening of the week.

Serves 4   **Preparation time:** 15 minutes   **Cooking time:** 20 minutes

250g/9oz dried thin egg noodles

1½ tbsp rapeseed/canola oil

500g/1lb 2oz skinless, boneless chicken breast, cut into thin strips

2 tsp grated ginger

2 garlic cloves, crushed

1 small onion, chopped

1 red pepper, deseeded and thinly sliced

150g/5oz mangetout/snow peas or sugar snap peas

1 large carrot cut into thin strips

1 large courgette/zucchini, cut into thin strips

150g/5oz baby corn

juice of 1 lime

2 tbsp sweet chilli sauce

1 tbsp soy sauce

80ml/2½fl oz/⅓ cup chicken stock

1 handful of coriander/cilantro leaves, chopped

1 Cook the noodles in a large saucepan of boiling water for 5 minutes, or until tender. Drain well, then toss with ½ tablespoon of the oil to prevent them sticking together. Leave to one side.

2 Heat the remaining oil in a non-stick wok or large frying pan over a high heat. Add about half the chicken so the wok is not overcrowded, and fry for 2–3 minutes, stirring, until browned. Using a slotted spoon, remove the chicken from the wok and cook the remaining chicken, then remove it from the wok.

3 Add the ginger, garlic and onion to the wok and stir-fry for 2 minutes, or until soft. Add the remaining vegetables and stir-fry for 3 minutes, or until tender but still crisp.

4 Add the lime juice, chilli and soy sauces and stock and bring to the boil. Add the noodles and toss to warm through. Return the chicken to the pan and reheat thoroughly. Sprinkle with the coriander/cilantro and serve hot.

Nutrition facts (per serving)   Calories 515   Carbohydrate 40g
Protein 34.2g   Fat 25.1g (of which saturates 5.7g)

Nepalese Chicken with Rice

This recipe was inspired by a trip to Nepal when I ran the Manaslu trail race. I was brought up with Indian flavours and I find it fascinating to see how a few changes to the spices or the cooking method can completely change a finished dish. The taste of this is superb – plus it is rich in lean protein and high in antioxidants.

Serves 4   Preparation time: 10 minutes, plus 30 minutes' marinating
Cooking time: 45 minutes

1 tsp turmeric
pinch of sea salt
1 tsp freshly ground black pepper
3 skinless chicken breasts, cubed
1 tsp mustard seeds
1 tsp fenugreek seeds
2 tbsp rapeseed/canola oil
2 garlic cloves, crushed
1 tbsp grated root ginger

2 dried red chillies, deseeded and
  finely chopped
1 tsp ground cumin
2 bay leaves
1 large onion, chopped
500ml/17fl oz/2 cups chicken stock
2 large tomatoes, chopped
150g/5½oz/¾ cup basmati rice
1 handful of coriander/cilantro
  leaves, chopped

1 Rub the turmeric, salt and pepper all over the chicken, cover and leave to marinate in the fridge for 30 minutes.

2 Put the mustard seeds in a frying pan over a medium heat and dry-roast for a few seconds, or until you can smell their aroma, being careful not to burn the spices, then tip them into a mortar or coffee grinder. Repeat with the fenugreek seeds. Crush to a coarse powder.

3 Heat the oil in a wok over a medium-high heat. Add the spice mixture, garlic, ginger, chillies, cumin and bay leaves and stir-fry for 20 seconds. Add the onion and sauté for 3–6 minutes until slightly translucent. Add the marinated chicken and stir-fry for 4 minutes, then add the stock and tomatoes. Bring to the boil, then turn the heat down to low and simmer for 35 minutes, or until the chicken is tender and the sauce has thickened.

4 Meanwhile, cook the rice in boiling water for 10 minutes, or until tender. Sprinkle the chicken with the coriander/cilantro and serve with the rice.

Nutrition facts (per serving) Calories 443 Carbohydrate 37.4g
Protein 36g   Fat 15.6g (of which saturates 3.7g)

Punjabi Chicken Biryani

A quick and easy way to spice up chicken for a mid-week meal, this Indian-inspired dish is really easy to make and has a lovely spicy taste.

Serves 4   **Preparation time:** 15 minutes   **Cooking time:** 1 hour

1 tbsp rapeseed/canola oil

1 tsp cumin seeds

1 large onion, chopped

2 garlic cloves, chopped

2.5cm/1in piece of root ginger, peeled
   and chopped

400g/14oz canned chopped tomatoes

1 tsp garam masala

½ tsp chilli powder

½ tsp turmeric

500g/1lb 2oz skinless chicken

250g/9oz frozen mixed
   vegetables, defrosted

120g/4¼oz/heaped ½ cup brown
   basmati rice

600ml/21fl oz/scant 2½ cups
   chicken stock

1 handful of coriander/cilantro
   leaves, chopped

low-fat plain yogurt and mango
   chutney, to serve

1 Heat the oil in a large saucepan over a medium heat. Add the cumin seeds and fry until you can smell their aroma, then add the onion, garlic and ginger and cook for about 5 minutes, stirring occasionally, until golden brown.

2 Add the tomatoes, garam masala, chilli powder and turmeric and cook for a few minutes, stirring occasionally, until the sauce becomes thick and slightly darker in colour.

3 Cut the chicken into chunks and cook for a few minutes until coated with the curry sauce. Add the vegetables and rice and cook for a further few minutes, stirring occasionally, until everything is well blended.

4 Pour the stock into the pan, cover and bring to the boil, then turn the heat down to low and simmer for about 45 minutes or until the chicken is cooked through, the rice is just tender and all the stock has been absorbed. You can add more boiling water to the saucepan as needed to ensure the chicken and rice are cooked.

5 Sprinkle with the coriander/cilantro and serve with yogurt and mango chutney.

Nutrition facts (per serving) Calories 487   Carbohydrate 40g   Protein 33g
Fat 9.2g (of which saturates 2.6g)

Char-Grilled Chicken Pasta Salad

After a hard workout on a long summer day, what better way to refuel than with this pasta salad? It is packed full of the slow-release carbohydrate and lean protein you need. Play around with the salad ingredients and come up with your own favourite combination.

Serves 4   **Preparation time:** 15 minutes   **Cooking time:** 15 minutes

320g/11¼oz/3½ cups wholegrain pasta
1½ tbsp rapeseed/canola oil
150g/5oz fine green beans, halved
500g/1lb 2oz skinless, boneless chicken breasts, cut into chunks
10cm/4in piece of cucumber, chopped

150g/5oz/heaped 1 cup sweetcorn/corn kernels, frozen or canned with no added salt and sugar
150g/5oz/1 cup cherry tomatoes, halved
3 tbsp fat-free plain yogurt
juice of ½ lemon
1 handful of chives, chopped

1 Cook the pasta in a large saucepan of boiling water for 8 minutes, or until tender. Drain well, then toss with ½ tablespoon of the oil to prevent the shapes sticking together. Leave to one side.

2 Meanwhile, cook the beans in a small saucepan of boiling water for 4 minutes, or until tender. Drain well and leave to one side.

3 Heat the oil in a griddle pan, add the chicken and fry for about 5 minutes, stirring occasionally, until cooked through. Leave to one side.

4 Mix the cucumber, sweetcorn/corn, tomatoes and green beans in a large salad bowl. Add the chicken and pasta and toss together gently.

5 Put the yogurt in a small bowl and mix in the lemon juice and chives. Add to the chicken salad and toss once more so that the yogurt dressing has mixed through. Serve straight away or cover with cling film/plastic wrap and keep in the fridge until ready to eat.

Nutrition facts (per serving) Calories 642 Carbohydrate 66.6g Protein 38g Fat 25.3g (of which saturates 5.6g)

Turkey Pesto Kievs

To make a change from chicken, this dish uses turkey as a lean protein source. It is also a healthier take on the traditional breaded chicken Kiev that can be bought in the shops. You can use shop-bought pesto but you might like to make your own from my recipe.

Serves 4   **Preparation time:** 15 minutes   **Cooking time:** 30 minutes

4 skinless, boneless turkey fillets
50g/1¾oz Mixed Nut Pesto (see page 256)
2 tsp clear honey
1 tsp rapeseed/canola oil
Roasted Mediterranean Vegetables (see page 256), to serve

1 Preheat the oven to 180°C/350°F/Gas 4.

2 Take each turkey fillet and make a slit lengthways, leaving one side uncut. Spread a quarter of the pesto inside each turkey fillet.

3 Mix together the honey and oil in a small bowl, then brush each fillet with the mixture. Bake for 25–30 minutes until the turkey is cooked and the juices run clear when pierced with the tip of a sharp knife. If the top starts to brown too quickly, cover with kitchen foil.

4 Serve with the roasted vegetables.

Nutrition facts (per kiev) Calories 225 Carbohydrate 3.7g Protein 28g
Fat 10.7g (of which saturates 2.8g)

Half & Half Chilli con Carne

Although athletes do not need to remove all fat from their diets, it is recommended that saturated fat is kept to a minimum. This recipe for chilli con carne halves the amount of beef and replaces it with lentils, which provide soluble fibre, iron and protein, while keeping overall fat intake fairly low. This dish can be served just on its own, if your training needs do not dictate the need for additional carbohydrates, but it also goes really well with a baked potato or boiled brown rice.

Serves 4   **Preparation time:** 20 minutes   **Cooking time:** 40 minutes

125g/4½oz minced/ground lean beef

1 tbsp rapeseed/canola oil

1 onion, chopped

1 garlic clove, crushed

400g/14oz canned chopped tomatoes

2 tsp yeast extract

1 tsp paprika

½ tsp chilli powder

1 tsp dried oregano

1 tsp dried herbes de Provence

1 tsp light soft brown sugar

1 large courgette/zucchini, sliced

150g/5½oz mushrooms, sliced

150g/5½oz broccoli

80g/2¾oz/⅓ cup red lentils

400g/14oz canned kidney beans, drained and rinsed

sea salt and freshly ground black pepper

1 Dry-fry the beef in a non-stick frying pan over a medium heat for about 5 minutes, stirring, until cooked through. Leave to one side.

2 Heat the oil in a large wok or frying pan over a medium heat. Add the onion and garlic and cook for 5 minutes, or until golden brown.

3 Add the tomatoes, yeast extract, paprika, chilli, oregano, herbes de Provence and sugar and cook for a few minutes, stirring, until blended. Add the beef, vegetables and lentils and cook for a few more minutes.

4 Pour in 400ml/14fl oz/generous 1½ cups water and season with salt and pepper. Bring to the boil over a high heat, then turn the heat down to low and simmer for about 20 minutes, stirring occasionally, until the lentils are tender and most of the liquid has been absorbed.

5 Stir in the kidney beans and heat through. Serve hot.

Nutrition facts (per serving) Calories 294 Carbohydrate 40g Protein 22g Fat 6.3g (of which saturates 1.3g)

Fruity Steak Stir-Fry

This meal is so quick and easy. You could even buy the ingredients on the way home from a training session! It is packed full of nutrients, including protein, carbohydrates, omega-3 fats and iron.

Serves 4   **Preparation time:** 10 minutes   **Cooking time:** 10 minutes

1 tbsp rapeseed/canola oil
1 garlic clove, crushed
300g/10½oz frying steak, cut into strips
150g/5½oz bag of mixed
    stir-fry vegetables

250g/9oz ready-to-cook rice noodles
2 tbsp sweet chilli sauce
juice of 1 lime
50g/1¾oz/heaped ⅓ cup raisins
50g/1¾oz/heaped ⅓ cup walnut halves

1 Heat the oil in a large wok over a high heat. Add the garlic, then the steak strips and stir-fry for a few minutes until cooked through.

2 Add the vegetables and noodles and stir-fry for about 3 minutes.

3 Add the chilli sauce, lime juice, raisins and walnut halves and stir-fry for a further 2–3 minutes, then serve straight away.

Nutrition facts (per serving) Calories 547 Carbohydrate 69.4g
Protein 26.2g Fat 18.9g (of which saturates 3.8g)

Roasted Aubergine & Beef Curry

Aubergines/eggplants are fat free and low in calories but high in fibre. Roasting gives them a real smoky flavour and this adds a great depth to this curry. By combining them with the beef in this dish, once again it reduces the overall saturated fat content while still providing good sources of protein and iron.

Serves 4   **Preparation time:** 5 minutes   **Cooking time:** 1 hour

2 large aubergines/eggplants

1 tbsp rapeseed/canola oil

1 large onion, chopped

2 garlic cloves, finely chopped

2 tbsp red curry paste

400g/14oz canned chopped tomatoes

300g/10½oz braising beef, diced

50g/1¾oz creamed coconut

sea salt and freshly ground black pepper

4 wholemeal pitta breads, warmed, to serve

1 Preheat the oven to 150°C/300°F/Gas 2.

2 Pierce the aubergines/eggplants through the skin in several places. Put on a baking sheet and bake for 20–30 minutes until the flesh is soft. Leave until cool enough to handle, then remove the skin and chop the flesh.

3 Heat the oil in a large wok over a medium-high heat, add the onion and garlic and fry for about 3 minutes until golden brown. Stir in the curry paste and cook until you can smell the aroma of the spices. Add the tomatoes and cook for a further few minutes until you have a nice thick, smooth sauce.

4 Add the aubergine/eggplant flesh, the beef and 400ml/14fl oz/generous 1½ cups water. Cover, bring to the boil over a high heat, then turn the heat down to low and simmer for about 20 minutes until both meat and vegetables are cooked through and most of the liquid has been absorbed.

5 Just before serving, season with salt and pepper to taste, spoon the creamed coconut over the top, then serve with warmed pittas.

Nutrition facts (per serving)   Calories 392   Carbohydrate 27.9g
Protein 27.6g   Fat 19.3g (of which saturates 10g)

Sausage Casserole

Although we should be reducing our overall intake of processed meat, including it occasionally is not a problem. Choose good-quality sausages – there is a huge range – or another option is you could, like me, use tofu-based sausages instead. I do like one-pot meals that can just be put in a slow cooker or in the oven and left to cook while you get on with other things. This meal is also a sneaky way of getting reluctant vegetable eaters to eat some veggies!

Serves 4   **Preparation time:** 15 minutes   **Cooking time:** 1 hour

8 lean sausages
400g/14oz canned chopped tomatoes
400g/14oz canned baked beans
1 large courgette/zucchini, cut
   into chunks
2 large carrots, cut into chunks
2 garlic cloves, finely chopped

4cm/1½in piece of root ginger, peeled
   and finely chopped
150g/5½oz fine green beans, halved
1 tsp paprika
1 handful of rosemary leaves
wholegrain toast, to serve

1 Preheat the oven to 180°C/350°F/Gas 4.

2 Put all the ingredients except the toast in a casserole dish and stir well. Cover and cook for about 1 hour until the sausages and vegetables are cooked.

3 Serve with wholegrain toast.

Nutrition facts (per serving) Calories 309 Carbohydrate 36.3g
Protein 22.7g Fat 9.4g (of which saturates 2.7g)

Chilli Chard & Pork Rice

This dish came about because we get a vegetable box delivered from a local farm and, during spring, there always seems to be an abundance of chard! Chard is very similar to spinach so is also high in folate, iron and nitrates.

Serves 4   **Preparation time:** 15 minutes   **Cooking time:** 20 minutes

1 tbsp rapeseed/canola oil
1 onion, thinly sliced
3 garlic cloves, finely chopped
500g/1lb 2oz pork fillets, cut into strips
120g/4¼oz/heaped ½ cup basmati rice
175g/6oz chard
1 small red chilli, deseeded and finely chopped
juice of 1 lemon
sea salt and freshly ground black pepper

1 Heat the oil in a large saucepan over a medium heat, add the onion and garlic and fry for about 4 minutes, stirring occasionally, until golden.

2 Add the pork strips and cook over a low heat for about 5 minutes until they are browned and tender.

3 Add the rice, chard, chilli and lemon juice to the pan, then pour in 500ml/ 17fl oz/2 cups water and season with salt and pepper. Bring to the boil over a high heat, then turn the heat down to low and simmer for about 8 minutes, stirring occasionally, until all the water has been absorbed.

4 Serve hot or leave to cool and serve cold.

Nutrition facts (per serving)   Calories 427   Carbohydrate 30g   Protein 35g Fat 18.1g (of which saturates 5.6g)

Purple Pancetta Penne

You can't get a better combination than purple sprouting broccoli and pasta. If you have completed a hard weights session and want some additional dairy protein, you could replace the toasted almonds with feta cheese. This dish can be served hot or cold.

Serves 4   **Preparation time:** 10 minutes   **Cooking time:** 20 minutes

300g/10½oz/3½ cups wholegrain penne pasta
1 tbsp rapeseed/canola oil
1 garlic clove, finely chopped
100g/3½oz pancetta
300g/10½oz purple sprouting broccoli heads
juice of ½ lemon
50g/1¾oz/heaped ¼ cup whole blanched almonds

1 Cook the pasta in a large saucepan of boiling water for 8 minutes, or until tender.

2 Meanwhile, heat the oil in a frying pan over a medium heat, add the garlic and cook for 1 minute, then add the pancetta and fry for about 3 minutes until crisp. Stir in the broccoli heads and lemon juice and cook for a further 3–5 minutes until the broccoli is tender but still crisp.

3 In a small frying pan, toast the almonds for a few minutes until golden.

4 Drain the pasta, then turn it into a serving dish. Add the broccoli and toss together gently. Sprinkle the toasted almonds over the top and serve hot or leave to cool and serve cold.

Nutrition facts (per serving) Calories 508 Carbohydrate 62g Protein 26g Fat 20.3g (of which saturates 3.8g)

Sweet & Sour Pork Chops with Sweet Potato

If you grew up in a house where the staple was meat, potato and two vegetables, then this dish should appeal. Sweet potatoes should be included in all athletes' diets as they are a great source of slow-release carbohydrate and provide the 'sweet' element of this dish, while the cooking apple serves as the 'sour'.

Serves 4   **Preparation time:** 15 minutes   **Cooking time:** 1¼ hours

1 tbsp rapeseed/canola oil

4 pork shoulder steaks

1 onion, chopped

2 garlic cloves, finely chopped

30g/1oz/¼ cup plain/all-purpose flour

450ml/16fl oz/scant 2 cups
    chicken stock

400g/14oz canned chopped tomatoes

½ tsp mixed/apple pie spice

½ tsp ground cinnamon

2 large sweet potatoes (about 600g/1lb
    5oz total weight), peeled and cut
    into cubes

1 cooking apple, such as a Bramley,
    peeled, cored and diced

sea salt and freshly ground
    black pepper

1 Preheat the oven to 180°C/350°F/Gas 4.

2 Heat the oil in a large frying pan over a high heat, add the pork steaks and fry for 5 minutes, or until browned on both sides. Transfer to a casserole dish.

3 Add the onion and garlic to the pan and fry for 3 minutes, or until golden brown. Sprinkle in the flour, then gradually stir in the stock, tomatoes and spices. Season with salt and pepper and bring to the boil.

4 Add the sweet potatoes and apple to the casserole dish with the pork. Pour the sauce over the top. Cover and bake for 1 hour, or until the meat and potatoes are tender. Serve hot.

Nutrition facts (per serving) Calories 481 Carbohydrate 50g Protein 25g Fat 20.4g (of which saturates 6.3g)

Coriander Lamb with Quinoa

I'm not a big fan of the term 'super food' but quinoa really is a super grain. Packed full of slow-release carbohydrate and protein, this dish is ideal as a recovery option.

Serves 4   **Preparation time:** 15 minutes   **Cooking time:** 20 minutes

1 tbsp coriander seeds
1 tbsp cumin seeds
1 tbsp olive oil
1 red chilli, deseeded and chopped
juice of ½ orange

400g/14oz canned chickpeas,
   drained and rinsed 100g/3½oz
   spinach leaves
125g/4½oz/⅔ cup quinoa
4 lamb chops, 50g/2oz each
1 litre/35fl oz/4 cups stock

1 Preheat the grill/broiler. Put the coriander and cumin seeds in a non-stick frying pan over a medium heat and toast until you can smell their aroma. Transfer to a pestle and mortar and grind to a powder. Blend in the oil, chilli and orange juice to make a paste.

2 Brush the spice mix liberally over the chops and grill/broil for 20 minutes, turning and basting regularly, or until the chops are cooked.

3 Meanwhile, put the spinach and quinoa in a large saucepan and pour in the stock. Bring to the boil over a high heat, then turn the heat down to low and simmer for 12 minutes until the quinoa is soft. Drain well, then stir in the chickpeas and warm through over a low heat.

4 Serve the chops hot on a bed of quinoa.

Nutrition facts (per serving) Calories 492 Carbohydrate 57.5g
Protein 35.5g Fat 13.8g (of which saturates 2.9g)

Lamb & Spinach Curry

Another spiced-infused, antioxidant-packed curry, this is lovely served with brown rice or wholemeal pitta breads.

Serves 4   **Preparation time:** 15 minutes, plus 30 minutes' marinating
Cooking time: 1¼ hours

2 garlic cloves

4cm/½in piece of root ginger, peeled and grated

1 small, very hot green chilli, deseeded and thinly sliced

2 handfuls of coriander/cilantro leaves

500g/1lb 2oz boneless shoulder of lamb, cut into 2cm/1in pieces

1 tbsp rapeseed/canola oil

1 onion, chopped

1 tsp paprika

½ tsp turmeric

½ tsp salt

4 tbsp fat-free Greek yogurt

400g/14oz baby spinach leaves

4 wholemeal pitta breads, to serve

1 Put the garlic, ginger, chilli and coriander/cilantro into a food processor and blend to a paste. Rub the paste into the lamb, then leave to one side for about 30 minutes to marinate.

2 Heat the oil in a large saucepan over a high heat and cook the onion for about 4 minutes until it is golden and crispy.

3 Add the lamb to the pan, turn the heat down to medium and stir in the paprika, turmeric and salt. Cover and cook for 10 minutes, stirring once or twice. The lamb should shed some water.

4 Add the yogurt 1 tablespoon at a time, stirring each one in before you add the next. Add the spinach and stir for a few minutes until it wilts. Make sure everything is well combined, then cover and turn the heat down as low as possible. Leave to cook for 50 minutes, stirring occasionally, until the lamb is tender.

5 Serve hot with wholemeal pitta breads.

Nutrition facts (per serving) Calories 495 Carbohydrate 35.2g
Protein 42.4g Fat 19.1g (of which saturates 6.4g)

Mushroom & Lamb Moussaka

This carbohydrate-free dish makes a satisfying meal on a rest or low-intensity training day, without leaving you feel hungry or deprived.

Serves 4   **Preparation time:** 25 minutes   **Cooking time:** 1 hour

2 large aubergines/eggplants, sliced
250g/9oz minced/ground lean lamb
1 tbsp rapeseed/canola oil
2 garlic cloves, finely chopped
250g/9oz chestnut
   mushrooms, chopped
800g/1lb 12oz canned chopped tomatoes
1 tsp paprika

1 tsp dried mixed herbs
2 tbsp plain/all-purpose flour
500ml/17fl oz/2 cups skimmed milk
100g/3½oz mozzarella cheese, grated
sea salt and freshly ground
   black pepper
mixed salad, to serve

1 Put the sliced aubergine/eggplant in a bowl of salted water for 10 minutes, then drain.

2 Brown the lamb in a non-stick frying pan over a medium-high heat, then remove from the pan, drain off any excess fat and leave to one side.

3 Add the oil to the pan and return to a medium heat. Add the garlic and fry for 3 minutes, or until golden brown. Add the mushrooms and cook for 5 minutes, or until the mushrooms are soft. Add the tomatoes, paprika and herbs and season with salt and pepper.

4 Preheat the oven to 180°C/350°F/Gas 4.

5 Return the lamb to the pan and cook for a further 5–10 minutes over a low heat, stirring occasionally, while you make the white sauce.

6 Put the flour in a small saucepan and stir in enough of the milk to make a paste. Put the pan over a low heat and whisk in the remaining milk, then stir until the mixture comes to the boil and thickens into a white sauce.

7 Layer the mushroom and lamb mixture alternately with the slices of aubergine/eggplant in an ovenproof dish, then top with the white sauce. Sprinkle the mozzarella over the top, then bake for 30–40 minutes until you can see the mixture bubbling around the sides. Serve hot with salad.

Nutrition facts (per serving) Calories 380   Carbohydrate 36g   Protein 26g
Fat 15.2g (of which saturates 7.7g)

Moroccan Lamb Stew

Another hearty one-pot meal packed full of vitamins and minerals, this time with the characteristic sweetness of North African cuisine.

Serves 4   **Preparation time:** 20 minutes   **Cooking time:** 1 hour 10 minutes

1 tbsp rapeseed/canola oil

300g/10½oz minced/ground lean lamb

1 large onion, chopped

300g/10½oz (prepared weight) peeled, deseeded and diced butternut squash

400g/14oz canned chopped tomatoes

400g/14oz canned chickpeas, drained and rinsed

50g/1¾oz/⅓ cup dried apricots, chopped

150g/5½oz/1 cup frozen peas

2 carrots, diced

750ml/26fl oz/3 cups chicken or vegetable stock

4cm/1½in piece of root ginger, peeled and finely chopped

1 tsp turmeric

1 tsp ground cinnamon

1 tbsp tomato purée/paste

sea salt and freshly ground black pepper

chopped mint leaves and fat-free Greek yogurt, to serve

1 Preheat the oven to 180°C/350°F/Gas 4.

2 Heat the oil in a large frying pan over a medium heat, add the lamb and onion and fry for about 5 minutes until the lamb has browned.

3 Meanwhile, mix all the remaining ingredients in a tagine or large casserole. Stir in the lamb mixture. Cover and bake for about 1 hour until the vegetables are cooked and majority of the stock has been absorbed.

4 Sprinkle with mint leaves and serve with Greek yogurt.

Nutrition facts (per serving) Calories 533 Carbohydrate 62.9g Protein 29.6g Fat 19.8g (of which saturates 7.1g)

Zesty Mackerel Fillets

Although fish is a common choice for most athletes looking for an easy, lean protein option, oily fish is often overlooked, and yet we should be aiming to consume one or two portions a week to ensure that we meet our omega-3 fat requirements. Mackerel has a strong flavour but combined with all these antioxidant-rich herbs and spices, it works beautifully, providing a well-balanced training meal. You could also serve it with brown rice instead of couscous, if you prefer.

Serves 4   **Preparation time:** 15 minutes   **Cooking time:** 25 minutes

4 mackerel fillets

4cm/1½in piece of root ginger, peeled and chopped

2 garlic cloves, finely chopped

1 red chilli, deseeded and finely chopped

300ml/10½fl oz/1¼ cups vegetable stock

200g/7oz/scant 1¼ cups couscous

juice of 1 lime

2 tbsp soy sauce

2 tbsp sweet chilli sauce

1 handful of coriander/cilantro leaves, chopped

1 Preheat the oven to 200°C/400°F/Gas 6.

2 Put the mackerel fillets in a single layer in an ovenproof dish. Sprinkle with the ginger, garlic and chilli, then cover with the vegetable stock. Bake for about 20 minutes, or until the fillets flake easily when tested with a fork.

3 After 15 minutes, put the couscous in a bowl and cover with boiling water. Leave to stand, stirring occasionally, until most of the water has been absorbed and the couscous is soft. Drain off any excess water.

4 When the fish is almost cooked, put the lime juice, soy sauce, sweet chilli sauce, ginger and coriander/cilantro in a small saucepan over a low heat.

5 Spoon the couscous onto serving plates and top with the mackerel fillets. Pour the mackerel cooking juices into the saucepan and heat through, then pour the zesty sauce evenly over the mackerel and couscous and serve.

Nutrition facts (per serving) Calories 443 Carbohydrate 43.5g
Protein 28g Fat 16.1g (of which saturates 3.3g)

Thai-Style Baked Fish with Stir-Fried Vegetable Rice

Oily fish not only provides vital omega-3 fats but is also a good source of calcium and vitamin D. There have been numerous studies in recent years linking low vitamin D levels with depression, obesity and increased risk of infection in athletes, especially through the winter months. A 100g/3½oz salmon fillet will provide you with 20g of protein and around 80 percent of your daily vitamin D requirements.

Serves 4   **Preparation time:** 15 minutes   **Cooking time:** 20 minutes

4 salmon fillets
zest and juice of 1 lime
1 garlic clove, finely chopped
1 small red chilli, deseeded
   and chopped
1 tbsp rapeseed/canola oil
1 lemongrass stalk, finely chopped
150g/5½oz baby corn

150g/5½oz mangetout/snow peas
   or sugar snap peas
150g/5½oz baby carrots
120g/4¼oz/heaped ½ cup brown rice
300ml/10½fl oz/1¼ cups vegetable stock
1 handful of coriander/cilantro
   leaves, chopped

1 Preheat the oven to 180°C/350°F/Gas 4.

2 Put each fish fillet on a piece of kitchen foil large enough to loosely wrap the fish. Sprinkle with the lime juice, garlic and chilli, then seal the parcels loosely.

3 Bake for 20 minutes, or until the fish flakes easily with a fork.

4 Meanwhile, heat the oil in a wok over a medium heat, add the lemongrass and fry for a minute until you can smell the aroma. Turn the heat up to high, add all the vegetables and stir-fry for 3 minutes.

5 Stir in the rice and pour over the stock. Bring to the boil, then turn the heat down to low and simmer for 15–20 minutes, stirring occasionally, until all the stock has been absorbed and the rice is cooked.

6 Serve the salmon on a bed of rice with the cooking juices spooned over the top. Sprinkle with lime zest and coriander/cilantro to serve.

Nutrition facts (per serving) Calories 437 Carbohydrate 36g Protein 39g
Fat 15.8g (of which saturates 2g)

Salmon Pasta Bake

This is a vitamin D, calcium and omega-3-enriched version of the humble tuna pasta bake that has probably been a staple in your cooking repertoire since you were a student! By adding the extra vegetables and wholemeal pasta, you introduce fibre, making it a complete meal for after training.

Serves 4   **Preparation time:** 15 minutes   **Cooking time:** 1¼ hours

300g/10½oz/3 cups dried wholegrain pasta
2 salmon fillets, 120g/4¼oz each
100g/3½oz/¾ cup frozen peas
100g/3½oz/¾ cup frozen sweetcorn/corn kernels

100g/3½oz fresh spinach leaves
2 tbsp plain/all-purpose flour
570ml/20fl oz/2⅓ cups skimmed milk
1 handful of mint leaves, chopped
1 handful of basil leaves, chopped
50g/1¾oz mature/sharp cheese, grated

1 Preheat the oven to 180°C/350°F/Gas 4.

2 Cook the pasta in a large saucepan of boiling water for 8 minutes, or until tender. Drain well, then leave to one side.

3 Meanwhile, put the salmon fillets in an ovenproof dish, cover with kitchen foil and cook in the oven for 10–15 minutes until the salmon flakes easily when tested with a fork. Remove from the oven and lift off the skin. Add the peas, sweetcorn/corn, spinach and cooked pasta to the salmon.

4 Put the flour in a small saucepan and stir in enough of the milk to make a paste. Put the pan over a low heat and whisk in the remaining milk, then stir until the mixture comes to the boil and thickens into a white sauce. Stir in the mint and basil leaves.

5 Pour the sauce over the fish and pasta. Sprinkle the cheese over the top and bake for about 40–45 minutes until the cheese is golden brown and the sauce is bubbling around the edges. Serve straight away.

Nutrition facts (per serving) Calories 509 Carbohydrate 74.3g Protein 35g Fat 10.3g (of which saturates 3.2g)

Baked Sea Bass with Rice Noodle Salad & Salsa

This makes a lovely meal for a warm summer evening. I have used sea bass but any white fish would work. Rice noodles have a lighter, less dense texture than egg noodles, making them ideal to toss into salads. You could increase the amount of vegetables here and remove the noodles if you wanted to have this as a main meal on a rest or low-intensity day when carbohydrates don't need to be included in large amounts.

Serves 4   **Preparation time:** 20 minutes   **Cooking time:** 20 minutes

4 sea bass fillets

2 tbsp lemon juice

2 garlic cloves, finely chopped

1 tbsp rapeseed/canola oil

1 carrot, cut into thin batons

100g/3½oz mangetout/snow peas

300g/10½oz ready-to-fry
  rice noodles

2 recipe quantities Tomato Salsa
  (see page 202), to serve

1 Preheat the oven to 180°C/350°F/Gas 4.

2 Put each fish fillet on a piece of kitchen foil large enough to wrap it into a loose parcel. Sprinkle with the lemon juice and garlic, then seal the parcels loosely. Bake for 20 minutes, or until the fish flakes easily when tested with a fork.

3 When the fish is almost cooked, heat the oil in a wok over a high heat. Add the carrot, mangetout/snow peas and rice noodles and stir-fry together for 3 minutes, or until tender.

4 Divide the noodles among serving dishes, put a sea bass fillet on top and spoon over the cooking juices. Serve hot with the Tomato Salsa.

Nutrition facts (per serving) Calories 245 Carbohydrate 20g Protein 24g Fat 6.2g (of which saturates 0.6g)

Easy Fish & Chips

I usually find after a hard race, all I really want is chips/fries. This is my body's way of replacing glycogen stores and electrolytes in the form of salt. This version always hits the spot and by serving the chips/fries with fish, you add protein to help with repair and recovery.

Serves 4   **Preparation time:** 15 minutes   **Cooking time:** 45 minutes

4 fillets of any white or oily fish
zest and juice of 1 lemon
2 large baking potatoes (about 570g/1lb
   4oz total weight), sliced into wedges
1 sweet potato, about 300g/10½oz, sliced
   into wedges
1 tbsp rapeseed/canola oil
½ tsp dried Italian herbs
sea salt and freshly ground
   black pepper

For the Mushy Peas:
300g/10½oz/heaped 3¼ cups
   frozen peas
1 tbsp fat-free plain yogurt

For the Lemon Mayonnaise:
2 tbsp fat-free plain yogurt
1 tbsp low-fat mayonnaise
juice of ½ lemon

1 Preheat the oven to 180°C/350°F/Gas 4.

2 Put the fish on a baking sheet and sprinkle with the lemon zest and juice.

3 Put the potato and sweet potato wedges on another baking sheet. Drizzle with the oil, sprinkle with the herbs and season with salt and pepper. Toss to cover them in the seasoned oil. Roast for 20 minutes, or until half cooked.

4 Turn the potatoes with a spatula, then put back in the oven. Put the fish in the oven at the same time and cook both for a further 20 minutes, or until the wedges are crisp and the fish flakes easily when tested with a fork.

5 Meanwhile, cook the peas in boiling water for about 3 minutes, then drain well. Blend the peas with the yogurt and 1 tablespoon water to produce a soft, mushy-pea texture.

6 Mix together the yogurt, mayonnaise and lemon juice to make the Lemon Mayonnaise.

7 Serve the fish, wedges and peas with the Lemon Mayonnaise.

Nutrition facts (per serving) Calories 471   Carbohydrate 61g   Protein 22g
Fat 16.8g (of which saturates 3.8g)

Magic Fish Pie

My children love this version of fish pie. In fact they don't seem to enjoy fish any other way! Once again, to save time, I have added vegetables to the main dish and also sneaked a few into the topping. This helps to reduce the carbohydrate content of the meal. The skimmed milk sauce, mixed fish and cheese topping make it an ideal choice after a hard strength and conditioning or weights session or a moderate workout.

Serves 4   **Preparation time:** 20 minutes   **Cooking time:** 1 hour

1 sweet potato (about 300g/10½oz), chopped

2 large carrots, chopped

1 large parsnip, peeled and chopped

670ml/23fl oz/2⅔ cups skimmed milk

60g/2oz low-fat cream cheese with chives

2 tbsp plain/all-purpose flour

1 smoked haddock fillet, cut into bite-size chunks

1 smoked mackerel fillet, cut into bite-size chunks

1 salmon fillet, cut into bite-size chunks

300g/10½oz mixed vegetables, such as frozen peas, sweetcorn/corn kernels and spinach

1 Preheat the oven to 180°C/350°F/Gas 4.

2 Put the sweet potato, carrots and parsnip in a large saucepan, cover with water and bring to the boil over a high heat. Turn the heat down to low and simmer for 10 minutes, or until tender. Drain, then mash with 100ml/3½fl oz/generous ⅓ cup of the milk and the cream cheese.

3 Put the flour in a small saucepan and stir in enough of the milk to make a paste. Put the pan over a low heat and whisk in the remaining milk, then stir until the mixture comes to the boil and thickens into a white sauce.

4 Put the fish pieces into the bottom of a large ovenproof dish and add the mixed vegetables. Pour the sauce over the top and stir together gently. Spread the mash mixture over the top.

5 Bake for 30–40 minutes until the pie is piping hot and the top is crisp. Serve straight away.

Nutrition facts (per serving) Calories 353 Carbohydrate 32g Protein 20g Fat 13.6g (of which saturates 5g)

Rosemary & Paprika Vegetable & Bean Hot Pot

I have to admit this is one of my favourite recipes. It is full of goodness from the vegetables, and the pulses add a good source of protein for vegetarians as well as iron, calcium and B vitamins. If you are planning on a moderate or hard training session the following day, or have just completed one, then serve the hot pot with toast or even a baked potato, but if it is a rest day, this is just as satisfying served alone as a chunky soup.

Serves 4   **Preparation time:** 15 minutes   **Cooking time:** 1 hour

2 garlic cloves, finely chopped

4cm/1½in piece of root ginger, peeled
   and chopped

2 large courgettes/zucchini, cut
   into chunks

2 large carrots, cut into chunks

200g/7oz broccoli florets

200g/7oz green beans, halved

400g/14oz canned chopped tomatoes

400g/14oz canned chickpeas, drained
   and rinsed

400g/14oz canned red kidney beans,
   drained and rinsed

1 tsp salt

2 tsp paprika

1 tsp soft light brown sugar

2 handfuls of rosemary leaves

sea salt and freshly ground
   black pepper

sourdough toast or baked potato,
   to serve (optional)

1 Preheat the oven to 180°C/350°F/Gas 4.

2 Put all the ingredients in a large casserole dish and pour in 400ml/14fl oz/generous 1½ cups water. Cover and bake for 1 hour, or until all the vegetables are cooked through and some of the juice has been absorbed.

3 Ladle into dishes and serve with slices of sourdough toast or a baked potato, if you like.

Nutrition facts (per serving without toast or potato) Calories 515
Carbohydrate 94g   Protein 30g   Fat 5g (of which saturates 0.4g)

Sweet Potato Risotto

An ideal choice before a long endurance day or race day, the protein in a traditional risotto has been removed and replaced with extra slow-release carbohydrate in the form of sweet potato to ensure that your glycogen stores are full. This dish also travels well, so if you are doing an event away from home and are able to reheat food, this is a good option to take with you.

Serves 4   Preparation time: 10 minutes   **Cooking time:** 20 minutes

300g/10½oz/1¾ cups basmati rice
2 sweet potatoes (about 600g/1lb 5oz
    total weight), peeled and chopped
750ml/26fl oz/3 cups vegetable stock
1 tbsp rapeseed/canola oil
1 garlic clove, finely chopped
2.5cm/1in piece of root ginger, peeled
    and finely chopped

250g/9oz stir-fry vegetables of
    your choice, such as baby corn,
    courgettes/zucchini and mangetout/
    snow peas/sugar snap peas
juice of 1 lime
1 tbsp sweet chilli sauce
1 tbsp soy sauce
1 handful of coriander/cilantro
    leaves, chopped

1 Put the rice and sweet potatoes in a large saucepan, pour over the stock and bring to the boil over a high heat. Turn the heat down to low and simmer for about 10 minutes until all the stock has been absorbed and both the rice and sweet potatoes are tender. Add a little more boiling water if necessary.

2 Heat the oil in a wok over a high heat. Add the garlic, ginger and vegetables and stir-fry for 3–5 minutes until the vegetables are tender but still crisp. Add the lime juice, chilli sauce and soy sauce. Stir in the rice and sweet potato mixture and stir-fry for a further 3 minutes until everything is hot and well mixed.

3 Serve hot, sprinkled with coriander/cilantro.

Nutrition facts (per serving) Calories 423 Carbohydrate 87g Protein 7g
Fat 4.1g (of which saturates 0.4g)

Butternut Squash & Coconut Curry

This is a good choice before a hard training session the following morning, or before an endurance event, if served with rice. However, if you just fancy a curry but you don't have a tough training session scheduled, then this also makes a hearty meal on its own.

Serves 4   **Preparation time:** 10 minutes   **Cooking time:** 15 minutes

1 tbsp rapeseed/canola oil

3 garlic cloves, finely chopped

1 red chilli, deseeded and finely chopped

2.5cm/1in piece of root ginger, peeled and finely chopped

1 tsp turmeric

6 cardamom pods, crushed

½ tsp ground cinnamon

400ml/14fl oz/generous 1½ cups low-fat coconut milk

400g/14oz butternut squash, peeled, deseeded and chopped into chunks

400g/14oz canned chickpeas, drained and rinsed

50g/1¾oz/½ cup ground almonds

1 tbsp lime juice

1 handful of coriander/cilantro leaves, chopped

sea salt and freshly ground black pepper

1 Heat the oil in a wok over a high heat. Add the garlic, chilli and ginger and stir-fry for 1 minute until you can smell their aroma. Add the turmeric, cardamom and cinnamon and stir-fry for 1 minute. Pour in the coconut milk and 150ml/5fl oz/scant ⅔ cup water. Bring to the boil, then turn the heat down to low and simmer for 5 minutes.

2 Stir in the butternut squash, chickpeas and ground almonds and continue to simmer for 10 minutes, or until the squash is tender.

3 Add the lime juice and coriander/cilantro, season with salt and pepper and serve straight away.

Nutrition facts (per serving)   Calories 603   Carbohydrate 57g   Protein 18g Fat 38g (of which saturates 23g)

Punjabi-Style Aloo Sabsi

Aloo sabsi is translated from the Punjabi as 'potato curry'. I grew up on this dish as a fussy child who did not like her vegetables! However, in recent years I have chosen to include this as a great option before an endurance event as it's a novel way of including more carbohydrate, especially if served with rice or chappatis. This dish can also be eaten cold, making it great as a portable snack on long bike rides, wrapped in a chappati or even in a wholemeal pitta bread.

Serves 4   **Preparation time:** 15 minutes   **Cooking time:** 25 minutes

1 tbsp rapeseed/canola oil

2 tsp cumin seeds

2 tsp black mustard seeds

1kg/2lb 4oz floury potatoes, such
   as Maris Piper, cut into chunks

400g/14oz canned chopped tomatoes

¾ tsp salt

1 tsp garam masala

¼–½ tsp chilli powder

½ tsp turmeric

juice of ½ lemon

1 Heat the oil in a large wok or balti dish over a high heat. Add the cumin and mustard seeds and stir-fry for 1 minute until you can smell their aroma. Add the potatoes and stir-fry for 3–5 minutes until coated with seeds.

2 Add the tomatoes, salt, garam masala, chilli powder, turmeric and lemon juice and mix together so the potatoes are covered in sauce and spices. Stir in 400ml/14fl oz/generous 1½ cups water. Cover and bring to the boil, then turn the heat down to low and simmer for 10–15 minutes until the potatoes are cooked and there is little juice left. Serve hot or cold.

Nutrition facts (per serving) Calories 221 Carbohydrate 44g
Protein 5.1g Fat 3.9g (of which saturates 0.8g)

Bulgar Wheat Curry

This is an excellent vegan recovery meal, although you don't need to be vegan to enjoy it. The combination of grain and pulses creates a whole protein with all the essential amino acids usually found in animal protein.

Serves 4   Preparation time: 15 minutes   Cooking time: 1 hour

1 tbsp rapeseed/canola oil

2 garlic cloves, finely chopped

1 onion, chopped

2 celery stalks, chopped

1 tsp ground cumin

1 tsp chilli powder

1 red pepper, deseeded
   and chopped

1 carrot, chopped

1 courgette/zucchini, chopped

400g/14oz canned kidney beans,
   drained and rinsed

400g/14oz canned aduki beans, drained
   and rinsed

125g/4½oz/⅔ cup bulgar wheat

1 handful of coriander/cilantro
   leaves, chopped

sea salt and freshly ground
   black pepper

1 Heat the oil in a large pan over a medium heat. Add the garlic and onion and fry for 3 minutes, or until golden brown. Add the celery, cumin and chilli powder and cook for a further 5 minutes, stirring regularly.

2 Add the pepper, carrot and courgette/zucchini and cook for 10 minutes, or until all the vegetables are tender. Add a little water if they start to stick to the pan.

3 Add both types of beans, the bulgar wheat and 500ml/17fl oz/2 cups water. Bring to the boil over a high heat, then turn the heat down to low and simmer for 30–40 minutes until the water has been absorbed.

4 Season to taste with salt and pepper and serve sprinkled with the coriander/cilantro.

Nutrition facts (per serving) Calories 361 Carbohydrate 61g Protein 19g
Fat 4.3g (of which saturates 0.8g)

Sweet Potato Parcels

The slow-release energy from sweet potatoes has been well documented for many years. This recipe is ideal for either before or after training. Feta is a lower-fat dairy option, which provides protein and calcium. Diets of individuals with high-calcium intakes from low-fat dairy sources have been linked with accretion of more lean muscle mass than in individuals with lower intake, making this dish a winning choice.

Serves 4   Preparation time: 5 minutes   **Cooking time:** 1 hour

4 sweet potatoes (about 1.2kg/2lb 12oz total weight)
1 bunch of spring onions/scallions, chopped
100g/3½oz feta cheese, crumbled
green salad leaves, cherry tomatoes and toasted seeds, to serve

1 Preheat the oven to 200°C/400°F/Gas 6. Pierce each sweet potato several times with a fork, then bake for 40–45 minutes until cooked through and tender. Remove from the oven and cut in half.

2 Preheat the grill/broiler to medium. Very carefully, use a spoon to scoop out the sweet potato flesh, keeping the skins intact. Mix the flesh with the spring onions/scallions and feta cheese, then spoon the mixture back into the empty skins.

3 Grill/broil the sweet potatoes for 5–10 minutes until golden brown. Serve with a tomato and toasted seed salad.

Nutrition facts (per serving) Calories 421 Carbohydrate 85g Protein 8g
Fat 5.8g (of which saturates 3.9g)

HERO FOOD: SWEET POTATO

Sweet potatoes have taken over in popularity from the humble white potato due to their high beta-carotene content and because they are a great source of complex carbohydrate, providing slow release energy and making it an ideal fuel before or after exercise. They are perfect baked and served with oily fish as a recovery meal or added to a risotto for a pre-endurance training meal. Add them to salads or make soup for great lunch options, helping to prevent that 4pm sugar slump. They are a must in every athlete's storecupboard.

Roasted Vegetable Tortilla Lasagne

Although pasta is the carbohydrate most often associated with athletes, it is not necessarily the most nutritious form. In this twist on traditional lasagne I use wholemeal tortillas instead to create a slow-release option. I have also boosted the vegetable content to make a dish that tastes indulgent but is packed full of micronutrients and dairy protein.

Serves 4   **Preparation time:** 15 minutes   **Cooking time:** 1¼ hours

2 aubergines/eggplants, sliced

2 courgettes/zucchini, sliced

1 red pepper, deseeded and cut into chunks

1 yellow pepper, deseeded and cut into chunks

300g/10½oz chestnut/cremini mushrooms

3 garlic cloves

300g/10½oz/2 cups cherry tomatoes, pierced

2 tbsp rapeseed/canola oil

1 tsp dried Italian herbs

1 tbsp plain/all-purpose flour

300ml/10½fl oz/1¼ cups skimmed milk

4 large wholemeal tortillas or wraps

50g/1¾oz mature/sharp Cheddar cheese, grated

sea salt and freshly ground black pepper

1 Preheat the oven to 180°C/350°F/Gas 4. Put all the vegetables, including the tomatoes, in a baking pan, sprinkle with the oil and herbs, season with salt and pepper and mix together. Roast for 30–40 minutes until the vegetables are tender and lightly browned.

2 Meanwhile, put the flour in a small saucepan and stir in enough of the milk to make a paste. Put the pan over a low heat and whisk in the remaining milk, then stir until the mixture comes to the boil and thickens.

3 Once the vegetables are cooked, spoon half of them into an ovenproof dish. Layer 2 tortillas over the top and then add the remaining vegetables. Top with the remaining 2 tortillas, pour over the sauce and sprinkle with the grated cheese. Return to the oven for a further 20–30 minutes until the cheese is golden. Serve hot.

Nutrition facts (per serving) Calories 471   Carbohydrate 65g   Protein 19g Fat 16.1g (of which saturates 5.8g)

Mixed Nut Pesto & Roasted Mediterranean Vegetable Pasta

I couldn't leave the pasta lovers out! This dish is suitable for vegans as the pesto is made without cheese. I have used coriander/cilantro leaves, but you could opt for the more traditional basil, if you prefer.

Serves 4   Preparation time: 15 minutes   **Cooking time:** 45 minutes

250g/9oz wholegrain pasta

½ tbsp rapeseed/canola oil

sea salt and freshly ground
   black pepper

For the Mixed Nut Pesto:

100g/3½oz/⅔ cup mixed
   unsalted nuts

1 tbsp tahini

100g/3½oz coriander/cilantro leaves

juice of 1 lemon

2 garlic cloves

**For the Roasted
   Mediterranean Vegetables:**

2 aubergines/eggplants, sliced

2 courgettes/zucchini, sliced

1 red pepper, deseeded and
   cut into chunks

1 yellow pepper, deseeded
   and cut into chunks

2 garlic cloves

300g/10½oz mushrooms

1 tbsp rapeseed/canola oil

1 tsp dried oregano

1 tsp dried Italian herbs

1 Preheat the oven to 180°C/350°F/Gas 4.

2 To make the pesto, put all the ingredients into a blender or food processor and pulse gently until the nuts have been broken down but the overall consistency of the pesto is still quite rough rather than a smooth paste.

3 Put all the vegetables onto a baking sheet. Sprinkle with the oil and herbs and toss together gently. Bake for 30–40 minutes until the vegetables are crisp and browned.

4 Meanwhile, cook the pasta in a large saucepan of boiling water for 10 minutes, or until tender. Drain well, then toss with the oil to prevent it from sticking together. Leave to one side.

5 Mix the pesto into the cooked pasta and serve hot.

Nutrition facts (per serving) Calories 538 Carbohydrate 73g Protein 21g Fat 21g (of which saturates 2.6g)

Italian Pasta

You could not have a sports recipe book without the simple traditional Italian tomato pasta dish. For some people this is all their stomachs can tolerate before a race. It is also something you can try before at home and is usually available if you are competing away. I have removed onion from this as it is well documented that onion is a gut irritant.

Serves 4   **Preparation time:** 5 minutes   **Cooking time:** 20 minutes

1 tbsp rapeseed/canola oil

3 garlic cloves, finely chopped

800g/1lb 12oz canned
   chopped tomatoes

1 tbsp tomato purée/paste

1 tsp dried oregano

2 tsp light soft brown sugar

1 large handful of basil leaves

360g/12¾oz/4 cups wholemeal pasta

sea salt and freshly ground
   black pepper

1 Heat the oil in a large frying pan over a medium heat, add the garlic and fry for 2–3 minutes until golden brown. Add the tomatoes, tomato purée/ paste, oregano and sugar and season with salt and pepper. Turn the heat up to high and bring to the boil, then turn the heat down to low and simmer for 10 minutes, stirring occasionally to remove any big lumps, or until the sauce is thick.

2 Stir in the basil leaves and cook for a further 2–3 minutes until the leaves have wilted.

3 Meanwhile, cook the pasta in a large saucepan of boiling water for about 10 minutes until tender. Drain well.

4 Pour the sauce over the pasta and stir well, then serve hot.

Nutrition facts (per serving) Calories 398 Carbohydrate 71g Protein 13g Fat 5.5g (of which saturates 0.8g)

SNACKS & PORTABLES

Dark Chocolate
& Ginger Muffins

I do not generally advocate cakes, biscuits/cookies, desserts and sweet
things. However, I have always believed that these foods can be included
in moderation in a healthy balanced diet. Muffins are easy to make and
I have reduced the fat and sugar content of these without affecting the
flavour. Serve them with a milk-based drink as a recovery option or take
them on bike rides, trail runs or hikes to keep energy levels topped up.

Makes 12 muffins   **Preparation time:** 15 minutes   **Cooking time:** 15 minutes

200g/7oz/1⅔ cups self-raising/
   self-rising flour
½ tsp baking powder
2 eggs, beaten
3 tbsp rapeseed/canola oil
100ml/3½fl oz/generous ⅓ cup
   skimmed milk
1 tsp vanilla extract

50g/1¾oz/heaped ¼ cup light soft
   brown sugar
75g/2½oz dark/bittersweet chocolate
   with ginger pieces, broken
   into chunks
2cm/¾in piece of root ginger, peeled
   and grated

1 **Preheat the oven to 180°C/350°F/Gas 4 and line a 12-hole muffin pan with
paper cases.**

2 **Sift the flour and baking powder together into a large bowl. Beat the eggs,
oil, milk, vanilla and sugar together in a separate bowl.**

3 **Gently fold the liquid mixture into the flour mixture but do not over-mix.
Add the chocolate chunks and grated ginger and fold together gently until
just combined.**

4 **Spoon the mixture into the prepared cases and bake for 15 minutes until
the muffins are well risen and the tops spring back when lightly pressed
with the fingertips.**

5 **Transfer to a wire rack to cool. Store in an airtight container for up
to 3 days.**

Nutrition facts (per muffin) Calories 155 Carbohydrate 20g Protein 3.3g
Fat 6.7g (of which saturates 2.1g)

Apple & Walnut Muffins

These are great to put in packed lunches for young athletes or even to enjoy with a cup of tea before a high-intensity training session. The use of walnut and walnut oil provides the additional bonus of omega-3 fats.

Makes 12 muffins   **Preparation time:** 15 minutes   **Cooking time:** 25 minutes

200g/7oz/1⅓ cups wholemeal or spelt self-raising/self-rising flour

4 eating apples, such as Cox's, peeled, cored and coarsely grated

75g/2½oz/heaped ½ cup walnuts, coarsely chopped

1 large egg

3 tbsp walnut oil

½ tsp vanilla extract

100ml/3½fl oz/generous ⅓ cup skimmed milk

60ml/2fl oz/¼ cup clear honey

1 Preheat the oven to 180°C/350°F/Gas 4 and line a 12-hole muffin pan with paper cases.

2 Put the flour in a large bowl. Stir in the grated apples and walnuts. Beat the egg, oil, vanilla, milk and honey together, then gently stir it into the apple mixture.

3 Spoon the mixture into the prepared paper cases and bake for 20–25 minutes until firm and golden.

4 Transfer to a wire rack to cool. Store in an airtight container for up to 3 days.

Nutrition facts (per muffin) Calories 166 Carbohydrate 26g Protein 5g Fat 5.7g (of which saturates 0.8g)

Carrot & Ginger Cake

Carrot cake is one of my favourites, so I modified the recipe so that it can also work as a great pre-training option. The wholemeal flour ensures that it is a good source of slow-release carbohydrate, while the blend of ginger and mixed spice give this cake real depth.

Makes 18 slices   **Preparation time:** 15 minutes   **Cooking time:** 1 hour

150ml/5fl oz/⅔ cup walnut oil, plus extra for greasing
6 eggs
150g/5½oz/heaped ¾ cup dark soft brown sugar
2 tsp mixed/apple pie spice
½ tsp vanilla extract

450g/1lb/3⅔ cups wholemeal self-raising/self-rising flour
500g/1lb 2oz carrots, grated
200g/7oz/1⅓ cups raisins
150g/5½oz/scant 1¼ cups walnuts
1cm/½in piece of root ginger, peeled and grated

1 Preheat the oven to 180°C/350°F/Gas 4 and grease a 20cm/8in cake pan.

2 Beat together the oil, eggs, sugar, spice and vanilla until well mixed. Fold in the remaining ingredients until just mixed.

3 Pour into the prepared cake pan and bake for 1 hour, or until a knife inserted in the centre comes out clean.

4 Transfer to a wire rack to cool. Store in an airtight container for up to 3 days.

Nutrition facts (per slice) Calories 257 Carbohydrate 36.5g Protein 8.3g Fat 9.5g (of which saturates 0.9g)

Courgette Tea Bread

This tea bread has a slight twist on the traditional recipe. I like to use fruit and vegetables in cakes whenever possible and this is no exception. This time I have used courgette/zucchini.

Makes 12 slices   **Preparation time:** 15 minutes   **Cooking time:** 30 minutes

3 tbsp rapeseed/canola oil, plus extra for greasing

85g/3oz/scant ⅓ cup clear honey

2 eggs

150ml/5fl oz/⅔ cup cooled chai tea

zest of 1 lemon

250g/9oz/1⅔ cups wholemeal spelt flour

1 tsp bicarbonate of soda/baking soda

¼ tsp baking powder

a pinch of salt

250g/9oz courgette/zucchini, grated

50g/1¾oz/ chopped mixed nuts

50g/1¾oz/heaped ⅓ cup raisins

a little butter, to serve

1 Preheat the oven to 180°C/350°F/Gas 4 and grease a 450g/1lb loaf pan.

2 Whisk together the oil, honey, eggs, tea and lemon zest until light and fluffy. Sift in the flour, bicarbonate of soda/baking soda, baking powder and salt, then gently fold it into the honey mixture. Swirl in the courgettes/zucchini, nuts and raisins but don't over-mix.

3 Pour into the prepared loaf pan and bake for 25–30 minutes until a knife inserted in the centre comes out clean.

4 Transfer the tea bread to a wire rack to cool. Slice and serve on its own or spread with a thin layer of butter.

Nutrition facts (per slice without butter)   Calories 127
Carbohydrate 16g   Protein 3g   Fat 6.9g (of which saturates 1.1g)

Sweet Potato Brownies

When I tell my athletes I have a recipe for brownies they are allowed to eat, their faces light up. This healthy version is low in fat and packed with slow-release carbohydrates in the form of sweet potatoes – a great snack to be eaten 1–2 hours before a training session or competition. Enjoyed with a glass of milk, they are also a good way to start replacing glycogen stores after a training session. Try replacing the cherries with dark chocolate chunks and walnuts for broken up brazil nuts, or experiment with your favourite dried fruit and nuts.

Makes 15 brownies   **Preparation time:** 15 minutes   **Cooking time:** 25 minutes

1 small sweet potato (about 225g/8oz)
100g/3½oz low-fat margarine
100g/3½oz dark/bittersweet chocolate,
   (at least 70% cocoa solids), broken
   into chunks
100g/3½oz/½ cup dark soft brown sugar
2 eggs

1 tsp vanilla extract
100g/3½oz/heaped ¾ cup plain/
   all-purpose flour
¼ tsp baking powder
50g/1¾oz/heaped ⅓ cup sour cherries
75g/2½oz/heaped ½ cup walnuts,
   roughly chopped

1 Preheat the oven to 200°C/400°F/Gas 6.

2 Pierce the potato with a fork and bake for 1 hour, or until soft. Leave until cool enough to handle, then scoop out the flesh into a bowl. You should have about 200g/7oz. While it is cooling, turn the oven down to 180°C/350°F/Gas 4 and line an 18cm/7in square cake pan with baking paper or kitchen foil.

3 Melt the margarine in a saucepan over a low heat, add the chocolate and stir until half melted, then remove from the heat and stir until melted.

4 Add the sugar to the sweet potato and beat until almost smooth. Stir in the margarine and chocolate, eggs and vanilla and beat until thick. Fold in the flour and baking powder, then the cherries and walnuts.

5 Spoon into the prepared pan, smooth the top and bake for 20–25 minutes until a crust forms on the top but the brownie is still soft under the crust. Leave to cool completely in the pan before slicing.

Nutrition facts (per brownie) Calories 172 Carbohydrate 20g
Protein 3.5g Fat 8.9g (of which saturates 2.7g)

Date Bars

Perfect for lunch boxes or for when you are on the move on a long bike ride or hike, these neat little bars are full of fast and slow-acting carbohydrate, as well as protein from the nuts and seeds, making them an almost virtuous sweet treat.

Makes 12 bars   **Preparation time:** 15 minutes   **Cooking time:** 30 minutes

3 tbsp rapeseed/canola oil, plus extra
   for greasing
100g/3½oz/⅔ cup pitted dates, chopped
80g/2¾oz/scant ⅓ cup clear honey
50g/1¾oz/heaped ⅓ cup mixed seeds

200g/7oz/2 cups rolled oats
75g/2½oz/heaped ½ cup chopped
   mixed nuts
50g/1¾oz/½ cup desiccated/dried
   shredded coconut

1 Preheat the oven to 150°C/300°F/Gas 2. Grease a 30 x 23 x 4cm/12 x 9 x 1½in baking pan and line it with baking paper.

2 Put the dates in a saucepan with 3 tablespoons water over a medium heat and bring to the boil. Turn the heat down to low and simmer for about 5 minutes until the dates are soft. Stir in the honey and oil over a low heat.

3 Meanwhile, put the seeds in a dry saucepan over a medium heat and toss for a few minutes until just beginning to brown. Tip into a large bowl and add all the remaining ingredients, then pour in the liquid mixture and stir well to combine.

4 Gently press the mixture evenly into the prepared baking pan, using a potato masher so that the mixture sticks together. Bake for 20–30 minutes until golden brown.

5 Leave to cool completely in the pan before until firm, then remove and cut into small bars.

Nutrition facts (per bar) Calories 228 Carbohydrate 26g Protein 5g
Fat 12.9g (of which saturates 3.9g)

Nut Butter Squares

These are little squares with a really high nutritional value as they contain carbohydrate, protein, essential fats, iron, vitamin E, magnesium and selenium. I take them on long hikes as an alternative to trail mix.

Makes 15 squares   **Preparation time:** 15 minutes, plus 1 hour setting

100g/3½oz/¾ cup Brazil nuts
2 tbsp smooth Nut Butter (see page 191), made with almonds
2 tbsp clear honey
1–2 tbsp skimmed milk powder
50g/1¾oz/heaped ⅓ cup chopped dried apricots
50g/1¾oz/heaped ⅓ cup raisins
25g/1oz/scant ¼ cup flaked/slivered almonds

1 Line a 20cm/8in cake pan with baking paper.

2 Put the Brazil nuts into a food processor and chop finely. Add the Nut Butter, honey, skimmed milk powder, apricots and raisins and blitz until they are all well combined and the mixture clumps together.

3 Tip the mixture into the prepared cake pan, smooth it into the corners and press down gently, then sprinkle with the flaked/slivered almonds. Put it into the fridge for about 1 hour to chill and firm up.

4 Turn the set cake onto a chopping board and cut into small chunks. Store in an airtight container in the fridge for up to 3 days.

Nutrition facts (per square) Calories 126 Carbohydrate 17g Protein 9g Fat 6.7g (of which saturates 1.2g)

Banana & Nut Butter Sandwich

Some flavours just go together naturally. Banana and nuts is one such combination, so I have brought them together here in this nourishing snack – perfect to accompany your recovery milkshake or smoothie.

Serves 1   Preparation time: 5 minutes

1 banana
2 tsp Nut Butter (see page 191) made with almonds, or nut butter of your choice

1 Slice the banana in half lengthways.

2 Spread the Nut Butter across one half of banana and then replace the top like a sandwich. This snack can be eaten straight away or wrapped and transported for later.

Nutrition facts (per serving) Calories 169 Carbohydrate 29g
Protein 3.4g Fat 6g (of which saturates 0.6g)

HERO FOOD: NUT BUTTER

Most athletes are surprised when I mention they can eat nut butters. Yes they are high in fat, but they are high in good fats and provide you with so many other essential nutrients, too, such as calcium, iron, magnesium, phosphorus and vitamin E. The high fat content means they help to keep you full and so can actually be useful for people who are trying to lose or watch their weight – but do be careful about quantity! Nuts also provide protein, so they can be particularly useful in vegan and vegetarian diets. One thing to watch, though – they don't make such a good choice post a high-intensity training session as the fat content means that it slows down the absorption of protein needed for recovery. One way round this is to have a glass of milk first (soya if you are vegan), and follow up with your nut butter!

Oatcakes

Oatcakes should be a staple in most athletes' cupboards, and although you can use shop-bought varieties, they are actually really easy to make. High in fibre and slow-release energy, they make the basis for a perfect pre- or post-training snack or even a light lunch. You can play around with flavours too – add ginger and sugar to make a sweeter version, or rosemary for a herby variety. They can be eaten with cheese or any of the dips in the book (see pages 269–71). I like to make a large quantity as they keep for two weeks in an airtight container.

Makes: 20 oatcakes   **Preparation time:** 15 minutes   **Cooking time:** 15 minutes

80g/2¾oz/heaped ¾ cup rolled oats
7g sachet/2 tbsp fast-action dried yeast
1 tsp sea salt
¼ tsp baking powder
3 tbsp olive oil

1 Preheat the oven to 180°C/350°F/Gas 4 and line two baking sheets with baking paper.

2 Put the oats in a food processor and grind to a fine flour. Add the yeast, salt and baking powder and pulse several times to mix together thoroughly. Add the oil and pulse until a dough starts to form.

3 Roll out the dough between two pieces of baking paper until it is about 5mm/¼in thick. Using a 2–3cm/¾–1¼in biscuit/cookie cutter, cut out rounds until there is no more dough. Re-roll and cut the trimmings.

4 Put all the oatcake rounds on the prepared baking sheets and bake for 15 minutes, or until they are light golden brown on the bottom.

5 Transfer to a wire rack to cool. Store in an airtight container for up to 2 weeks.

Nutrition facts (per oatcake)   Calories 33   Carbohydrate 3g
Protein 0.5g   Fat 2.4g (of which saturates 0g)

Pepper & Yogurt Dip

This is originally my mum, Katy's recipe. My mum has been a huge inspiration to me in many ways and has definitely influenced my culinary skills. She is an amazing cook and has taught me the importance of patience and using spice skilfully! This recipe is fantastic as a high-protein vegetarian dip alternative to hummus. Additionally it is a good way to use up yogurt that has gone slightly sour.

Serves 6   **Preparation time:** 5 minutes, plus chilling   **Cooking time:** 15 minutes

2 tsp rapeseed/canola oil
1 tsp black mustard seeds
1 green pepper, deseeded and chopped
1 red pepper, deseeded and chopped
30g/1oz/heaped ¼ cup gram (chickpea) flour
500g/1lb 2oz/2 cups fat-free plain yogurt

1 Heat the oil in a non-stick frying pan over a medium heat. Add the mustard seeds and fry for 1 minute, or until they start popping. Add the peppers and cook for 5 minutes, or until soft.

2 Stir in the gram flour and cook for 2 minutes, stirring continuously, until the flour has blended into the peppers. Turn the heat up to medium, add the yogurt and bring to the boil, then turn the heat down to low and simmer for about 5 minutes until the yogurt has a thick and paste-like consistency.

3 Transfer to a bowl and leave to cool, then cover with cling film/plastic wrap and chill in the fridge. Store for up to 5 days.

Nutrition facts (per serving) Calories 113 Carbohydrate 10g Protein 5g Fat 5.5g (of which saturates 1.2g)

Mackerel Pâté

Mackerel is an oily fish and therefore an excellent source of omega-3 fats, calcium and vitamin D. The cream cheese and yogurt soften its strong flavour and make this a nutritious topping for your Oatcakes (see page 268) and Black Pepper Pitta Crisps (see page 274), or even a great wrap filling.

Serves 4　**Preparation time:** 5 minutes

2 peppered smoked mackerel fillets, skinned
2 tbsp low-fat cream cheese
2 tbsp fat-free Greek yogurt
juice of 1 lemon
oatcakes (see page 268), to serve

1　Put all the ingredients in a food processor and pulse until smooth.

2　Spoon into a bowl, cover with cling film/plastic wrap and chill in the fridge before serving. It will keep for up to 2 days.

Nutrition facts (per serving)　Calories 181　Carbohydrate 1.6g　Protein 10g Fat 14.7g (of which saturates 4.5g)

Harissa & Cumin Hummus

Chopped carrots dipped in hummus are pretty well unbeatable as a great mid-afternoon pick-me-up, and although you can buy hummus from the shop, I wanted to demonstrate just how easy it is to make.

Serves 4   **Preparation time:** 10 minutes   **Cooking time:** 2 minutes

1 tsp cumin seeds
400g/14oz canned chickpeas, drained and rinsed
1 tbsp extra virgin olive oil
juice of 1 lemon
1 tbsp tahini
1 tsp harissa
sea salt

1 Put the cumin seeds in a dry saucepan over a medium heat and toss for a few minutes until just beginning to brown.

2 Tip the toasted seeds into a blender and add the remaining ingredients and 2 tablespoons water. Pulse until blended to the texture you prefer. I prefer chunkier hummus but if you want a smoother option, then add a little more water and pulse for longer.

3 Spoon into a bowl, cover with cling film/plastic wrap and chill in the fridge for up to 2 days.

Nutrition facts (per serving) Calories 125   Carbohydrate 11.4g
Protein 5.4g   Fat 6.7g (of which saturates 0.7g)

Spinach & Parmesan Muffins

These muffins are great as an alternative to a sandwich for lunch, as an accompaniment to soup for a light meal or even to keep up your energy on a long bike ride, trail run or hike instead of the usual sweet options on offer.

Makes 12 muffins   **Preparation time:** 15 minutes   **Cooking time:** 15 minutes

a little rapeseed/canola oil,
   for greasing
125g/4½oz spinach leaves, chopped
150g/5½oz/scant 1¼ cups plain/
   all-purpose wholemeal flour
1 tsp baking powder
a pinch of sea salt and freshly ground
   black pepper

2 eggs
80ml/2½fl oz/⅓ cup skimmed milk
3 tbsp white wine vinegar
2 tbsp olive oil
100g/3½oz Parmesan or mature/sharp
   Cheddar cheese, finely grated

1 Preheat the oven to 220°C/425°F/Gas 7 and grease a 12-hole muffin pan.

2 Put the spinach in a steamer over a saucepan of boiling water, cover and steam for 2 minutes until wilted. Drain and leave to one side.

3 Mix together the flour, baking powder and salt in a large bowl and season with pepper. Add the eggs, milk, vinegar and oil and stir until just combined. Fold in the spinach and grated cheese but do not over-mix.

4 Spoon the mixture into the prepared muffin pan and bake for 15 minutes, or well risen and slightly springy to the touch.

5 Transfer to a wire rack to cool slightly, then serve warm or cold. Store in an airtight container for up to 3 days.

Nutrition facts (per muffin) Calories 98 Carbohydrate 7.8g Protein 5.6g Fat 5.1g (of which saturates 1.8g)

Cheese & Chilli Scones

These lightly spiced scones are great served with soup or even a casserole or stew. They are good for lunch boxes and make a nutritious alternative to sweet bars and cakes on long endurance-training sessions.

Makes 12 scones   **Preparation time:** 20 minutes   **Cooking time:** 12 minutes

low-calorie cooking oil spray, for greasing

350g/12oz/2¾ cups self-raising/self-rising wholemeal flour, plus extra for dusting

1 tsp baking powder

½ tsp salt

3 tbsp rapeseed/canola oil

50g/1¾oz mature/sharp Cheddar cheese, grated

1 tsp dried chilli/hot pepper flakes

100g/3½oz/scant ½ cup fat-free Greek yogurt

100ml/3½fl oz/scant ½ cup skimmed milk

1 Preheat the oven to 220°C/425°F/Gas 7 and lightly grease a large baking sheet.

2 Put the flour, baking powder, salt and oil in a bowl and bring together until the mixture resembles breadcrumbs. Stir in the cheese and chilli/hot pepper flakes and make a well in the centre. Add the yogurt and half the milk and bring the mixture together to produce a soft dough.

3 Turn the dough out onto a lightly floured surface and shape into a ball, then roll out to about 2cm/¾in thick. Cut into 12 rounds using a 6cm/2½in biscuit/cookie cutter, lightly re-rolling the trimmings until all the dough has been used.

4 Put the scones on the prepared baking sheet and brush the tops with the remaining milk. Bake for 10–12 minutes until risen and golden in colour.

5 Transfer to a wire rack to cool. Store in an airtight container for up to 3 days.

Nutrition facts (per scone) Calories 136 Carbohydrate 17g Protein 5g Fat 5.4g (of which saturates 1.6g)

Black Pepper Pitta Crisps

The idea for these crisps originated one evening as my daughter was having a sleepover and I did not want them eating high fat/salt tortilla chips or crisps. They can be eaten on their own or with dips as a more substantial snack. And you can play around with the flavours – I have added garlic and salt and even soy sauce and chilli with great success.

Serves 4   **Preparation time:** 5 minutes   **Cooking time:** 5 minutes

4 wholemeal pitta breads
1 tbsp olive oil
freshly ground black pepper

1 Preheat the oven to 150°C/300°F/Gas 2.

2 Cut each pitta bread into at least 6 triangles and put them on a baking sheet. Brush with olive oil and sprinkle with pepper. Bake for 3–5 minutes until crisp.

3 Transfer to a wire rack to cool.

Nutrition facts (per serving) Calories 185 Carbohydrate 28g Protein 6g Fat 4.3g (of which saturates 0.7g)

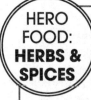

HERO FOOD: HERBS & SPICES

Herbs and spices are a great way to make even the most basic dish a little more interesting; who wouldn't prefer rosemary infused baked potato wedges over just potato wedges? Or how about the warming properties of ginger when blended with butternut squash for a hearty soup; and you really can't beat the blend of lime, chilli and coriander to add zest and flavour to a stir fry. However it is not just their ability to perk up meals that makes them so important to our daily diets. They are actually very potent and powerful antioxidants and a great way to ensure your immune system gets a boost.

Easy Snack Suggestions

Sometimes it is not possible to make all your own portable snacks or recovery options, so here are a few ideas for products that you can buy or make very quickly to help with your overall training nutrition.

Flavoured milk – any flavour

Milk-based drinks, such as lattes

Cereal bars – there are many on the market but some are better than others. The ones I tend to recommend to my athletes are:

> **Chia Charge bars** (from www.running food.co.uk)
> **9 bars** – all varieties (from most supermarkets and health food shops)
> **Naked bars** – all varieties (from most supermarkets and health-food stores)
> **Nookie bars** (from www.nookiebar.com)

Clif bars and shots

Dried fruit and nut mixes

Salted peanuts

Stuffed dates – try putting a teaspoon of low-fat cream cheese in a date as a quick, energy-rich snack

Jelly Babies

Gels – good options include TORQ, Clif or SiS, but most important is using ones you can tolerate.

RECOVERY DRINKS

Often after a hard training session, appetites can actually be suppressed at first, but it is also the most important time to take in nutrients to help with the recovery process. Having a drink could be the best solution as not only will it start replacing carbohydrate and protein, it will also help with rehydration. The general rule of thumb for a recovery drink is that it should be 3:1 carbohydrate to protein. The easiest way to achieve this is to use a milk-based option. A lot of the protein shakes and recovery drinks on the market are actually just glorified milk. Why not save some money and make your own tastier versions such as those included in this section? To make the perfect latte all you need is 1 shot of strong espresso topped with 250ml/9fl oz/1 cup warm milk.

Tropical Smoothie

This is so easy to make, but I usually suggest to my athletes that they have it ready in the fridge so they can drink it as soon as they get back from training – or you can have the ingredients waiting in a blender ready to turn on as soon as you step through the door! The Greek yogurt ensures that recovery protein requirements are met.

Serves 1   **Preparation time:** 5 minutes

200ml/7fl oz/¾ cup tropical fruit juice
200g/7oz/¾ cup fat-free Greek yogurt
1 handful of ice

1 **Put all ingredients in a blender and blend until smooth. Pour into a glass and serve straight away.**

Nutrition facts (per serving) Calories 239 Carbohydrate 38g Protein 20g
Fat 0g (of which saturates 0g)

Mocha Shake

One of my favourite recovery drinks, especially after a tough session on a hot day. Coconut water is known for its rehydration properties.

Serves 1   **Preparation time:** 5 minutes

3 tsp unsweetened cocoa powder
1 tsp sugar
1 tsp instant coffee powder
300ml/10½fl oz/1¼ cups skimmed milk
200ml/7fl oz/¾ cup coconut water
1 handful of ice

1 Put all ingredients into a blender and blend until smooth. Pour into a glass and serve straight away.

Nutrition facts (per serving)   Calories 140   Carbohydrate 25g
Protein 10g   Fat 0g (of which saturates 0g)

Recovery Hot Chocolate

This indulgent drink contains the right balance of carbohydrate and protein for recovery. It's amazing after a cold, late training session.

Serves 1   **Preparation time:** 5 minutes   **Cooking time:** 5 minutes

300ml/10½fl oz/1¼ cups skimmed milk
25g/1oz skimmed milk powder
20g/¾oz dark/bittersweet chocolate (at least 70% cocoa solids), broken into chunks

1 Put the milk and milk powder in a saucepan over a low heat, stirring occasionally, until the powder has dissolved into the milk. Add the chocolate and keep stirring until the chocolate has melted.

2 Pour into a mug and serve straight away.

Nutrition facts (per serving)   Calories 290   Carbohydrate 39g   Protein 19g
Fat 6.1g (of which saturates 4.3g)

DESSERTS

Frozen Vanilla Yogurt

Most of us feel the need for a sweet treat after a main meal. This recipe helps you meet your calcium requirements and daily protein intake – as well as being delicious.

Serves 4   **Preparation time:** 10 minutes, plus at least 4 hours' freezing

600g/1lb 5oz fat-free Greek yogurt
1 tsp vanilla extract
2 tbsp clear honey
1 vanilla pod/bean, split lengthways and seeds scraped out

1 Put the yogurt, vanilla extract and honey in a large bowl and stir in the vanilla seeds. Spoon the mixture into a 450g/1lb loaf pan, cover with cling film/plastic wrap and put in the freezer for at least 4 hours. Alternatively, you can freeze the yogurt in individual pots.

2 Take out of the freezer 10–15 minutes before serving to allow the dessert to soften.

Nutrition facts (per serving) Calories 121 Carbohydrate 15g Protein 16g Fat 0g (of which saturates 0g)

Frozen Peach Yogurt

This dessert offers an alternative flavour to vanilla but one that is still just as nutritious and a really great sweet treat to offer friends and family. The Greek yogurt makes it a high-protein choice.

Serves 4 **Preparation time:** 5 minutes, plus at least 4 hours' freezing

600g/1lb 5oz fat-free Greek yogurt
150g/5½oz fresh or frozen, defrosted peaches, pitted and chopped
2 tbsp clear honey

1 Put all the ingredients into a large bowl and stir until well blended.

2 Spoon the mixture into four freezer containers and freeze for at least 4 hours.

3 Remove from the freezer 10–15 minutes before serving to allow the dessert to soften.

Nutrition facts (per serving) Calories 133 Carbohydrate 18g Protein 16g
Fat 0g (of which saturates 0g)

HERO FOOD: GREEK YOGURT

I'm a great fan of yogurt as a recovery option, but I particularly favour fat-free Greek yogurt because of its high protein content. Most plain Greek yogurt provides 10g of protein per 100g/3½oz yogurt, which is double the amount found in standard yogurts. Protein is an important nutrient required in the recovery process in order to repair and rebuild muscles, helping them to adapt to the training process. Greek yogurt is an ideal choice due to its versatility – it can be mixed into fruit, added to smoothies, or eaten with cereal such as muesli or granola. You can also use it as a base for a slightly more decadent dessert, meaning you can enjoy your pudding guilt free, knowing that it is also the perfect recovery food.

Berry & Toasted Almond Pots

I like having friends over for dinner but I still see this an as opportunity to fuel my training correctly, which is why I came up with this recipe. It delivers on taste, looks beautiful and also continues to work as training food for me!

Serves 4   **Preparation time:** 10 minutes, plus cooling
Cooking time: 10 minutes

50g/1¾oz/heaped ⅓ cup flaked/slivered almonds
500g/1lb 2oz mixed berries, fresh or frozen, defrosted
400g/14oz fat-free Greek yogurt
4 heaped tsp clear honey

1 Put the flaked/slivered almonds in a dry frying pan over a medium heat and toss for a few minutes until just beginning to brown. Tip out and leave to one side.

2 Put the berries in a saucepan with 4 tablespoons water over a medium heat, bring to the boil, then turn the heat down to low and simmer for 10 minutes, or until the berries are soft and cooked with some juice remaining. Leave to cool slightly.

3 Spoon the berries into tall glasses or ice-cream bowls. Spoon the yogurt over the top, then drizzle 1 teaspoon honey over the top of each portion. Top each bowl with some toasted flaked/slivered almonds and serve. This dessert can also be kept in the fridge until ready to serve.

Nutrition facts (per serving) Calories 241 Carbohydrate 27g Protein 15g
Fat 8.7g (of which saturates 0.6g)

Summer Fruit & Mint Kebabs

These are a great way to enjoy summer fruits. They also showcase
a variety of colours, ensuring that you are taking on more nutrients.
Make enough for the whole family and put them in lunch boxes.

Serves 4   **Preparation time:** 15 minutes

250g/9oz strawberries, hulled and halved
1 melon, peeled, pitted and cubed
1 handful of mint leaves
3 tbsp orange juice

1 **Thread the strawberry halves, melon cubes and mint leaves alternately
on eight kebab skewers, leaving enough room at one end to hold the kebab.
Brush with the orange juice.**

2 **Serve straight away or transfer to an airtight container to be
enjoyed later.**

Nutrition facts (per serving)   Calories 63   Carbohydrate 15g   Protein 1.4g
Fat 0g (of which saturates 0g)

Mango & Kiwi Baskets

A tropical twist to a standard fruit salad here – be inventive and try other combinations of fruit, like pineapple and pear or grapes and melon.

Serves 4   **Preparation time:** 10 minutes

2 large mangoes, peeled and pitted
2 kiwis, peeled and chopped
4 tbsp low-fat tropical fruit yogurt

1 Cut the mango flesh out of the skin, trying to keep the skin of each mango half intact. Chop the flesh and mix it with the kiwis, then spoon the fruit back into the mango skins, arranging any extra fruit around the shells.

2 Serve with a spoonful of yogurt.

Nutrition facts (per serving)   Calories 110   Carbohydrate 24g   Protein 3.5g Fat 0g (of which saturates 0g)

Nectarine Compôte with Zesty Crème Fraîche

The combination of flavours in this fruit-based dessert make it a decadent and yet guilt-free post-dinner sweet treat.

Serves 4   **Preparation time:** 10 minutes, plus 10 minutes' cooling
Cooking time: 15 minutes

4 large, ripe nectarines, quartered and pitted
zest and juice of 1 orange
1 tbsp dark soft brown sugar
1 tsp grated root ginger
120g/4¼oz/½ cup low-fat crème fraîche

1 Put the nectarines, orange juice, sugar and ginger in a saucepan with 3 tablespoons water over a low heat and cook gently for 10 minutes, or until the nectarines are soft.

2 Lift out the nectarine quarters into bowls, using a slotted spoon, leaving the juice in the saucepan. Bring to the boil, then turn the heat down to low and simmer for a few minutes until the juice is syrupy.

3 Remove from the heat and stir to allow the mixture to cool slightly, then stir in the crème fraîche and mix with the nectarines. Sprinkle over the orange zest and serve.

Nutrition facts (per serving) Calories 144 Carbohydrate 22g Protein 1.2g
Fat 4g (of which saturates 4g)

Fruity Fool

Fruit is naturally sweet, which is why it makes such a great base for desserts. Plus it is also very versatile, as shown in this chapter. Berries, in particular, have a beneficial property in that they help regulate blood sugar levels and also cause vaso-dilation, which aids blood flow, subsequently reducing blood pressure.

Serves 4   **Preparation time:** 15 minutes, plus chilling
Cooking time: 8 minutes

300g/10½oz mixed fruit, such as raspberries, blackberries,
    blueberries or currants
55g/2oz/¼ cup caster/granulated sugar
150g/5½oz/heaped ½ cup low-fat crème fraîche
150g/5½oz/heaped ½ cup fat-free plain yogurt

1 Reserve about 55g/2oz of the mixed fruit for decoration. Put the remaining mixed fruit in a saucepan with 2 tablespoons water over a high heat. Bring just to the boil, then turn the heat down and cook gently for 5 minutes, or until soft and very juicy. Stir in the sugar until dissolved.

2 Remove from the heat and leave to cool slightly. Pour into a food processor or blender and purée. Set aside to cool completely.

3 Whisk the crème fraîche, using an electric mixer, until thick. Add the yogurt and whip into the mixture, then mix in the cooled fruit purée.

4 Spoon into dessert dishes or goblets and chill for several hours. Top with the reserved fruit before serving.

Nutrition facts (per serving)   Calories 187   Carbohydrate 27g   Protein 2.6g
Fat 6.1g (of which saturates 5.3g)

Berry Meringues

These seem to be a hit with adults and children alike and offer you a simple and quick way to make strawberries a bit more exciting.

Serves 4   **Preparation time:** 5 minutes

4 meringue nests
250g/9oz strawberries, hulled and chopped
4 scoops of Frozen Vanilla Yogurt (see page 280)

1 Put the meringue nests on serving plates and divide the chopped strawberries between them – don't worry if some are tumbling over the sides. Top with a scoop of Frozen Vanilla Yogurt and serve.

Nutrition facts (per serving)   Calories 160   Carbohydrate 30g
Protein 11.4g   Fat 0g (of which saturates 0g)

Greek-Style Potted Lemon Cheesecake

If you are following a strict training plan and trying to fuel accordingly, standard cheesecake would be difficult to validate. However, this makes a much lighter option, with the added benefits of being high in protein, essential fatty acids, vitamin E, calcium, phosphorus and magnesium.

Serves 4   Preparation time: 10 minutes

4 tbsp Nut Butter, made with almonds (see page 191)
zest and juice of ½ lemon
4 tsp lemon curd
400g/14oz fat-free Greek yogurt

1 Put 1 tablespoon Nut Butter at the bottom of four individual dessert bowls, tall glasses or goblets.

2 In a large bowl, mix together the lemon juice, lemon curd and yogurt until well blended. Layer this yogurt mix over the top of each almond butter base and smooth the top. Sprinkle with the lemon zest, cover and chill in the fridge until ready to serve.

Nutrition facts (per serving) Calories 179 Carbohydrate 8.2g Protein 14g Fat 11g (of which saturates 1.9g)

Lemon Drizzle Polenta Cake

Although I enjoy fruit-based desserts, sometimes we all just need a bit more. This cake is light and fresh and a great alternative when all you want is something sweet and stodgy!

Makes 12 slices **Preparation time:** 15 minutes **Cooking time:** 40 minutes

80ml/2½fl oz/⅓ cup rapeseed/canola oil, plus extra for greasing
175g/6oz/1⅓ cups self-raising/self-rising flour
1½ tsp baking powder
50g/¾oz/½ cup ground almonds
50g/1¾/½ cup polenta/cornmeal
finely grated zest and juice of 2 lemons
115g/4oz/scant ½ cup golden caster/raw cane sugar
2 large eggs
225g/8oz/scant 1 cup plain yogurt

1 Heat the oven to 180°C/160°C/Gas 4. Lightly grease a 20cm/8in deep cake pan and line the base with baking parchment.

2 For the cake, put the flour, baking powder, ground almonds and polenta/cornmeal in a large mixing bowl. Stir in the lemon zest and sugar, then make a well in the centre.

3 Beat the eggs in a bowl, then stir in the yogurt. Tip this mixture into the dry ingredients, along with the oil and lemon juice, then briefly and gently stir with a large metal spoon so everything is just combined, without over-mixing.

4 Spoon the mixture into the prepared pan and level the top. Bake for 40 minutes, or until a skewer inserted in the centre comes out clean. Cover the cake loosely with foil for the final 5–10 minutes if it starts to brown too quickly.

5 Let the cake cool in the pan for a few minutes, then transfer to a wire rack to cool.

Nutrition facts (per slice) Calories 211 Carbohydrate 27.5g Protein 4.5g Fat 9.6g (of which saturates 1g)

Rhubarb Granola Crumble

Fruit crumble is a favourite with many people. This recipe removes the stodgier, higher-fat traditional topping and replaces it with a slow-release carbohydrate option, which is useful when aiming to fuel up for an endurance or high-intensity session the following morning.

Serves 4   **Preparation time:** 15 minutes   **Cooking time:** 10 minutes

4–6 rhubarb stalks, cut into small chunks
1 tbsp caster/granulated sugar
1 tsp mixed/apple pie spice
60g/2¼oz/½ cup Granola (see page 184)

1 Preheat the oven to 150°C/300°F/Gas 2.

2 Put the rhubarb and sugar in a saucepan with about 3 tablespoons water and cook over a low heat for about 8 minutes, or until the rhubarb is soft. Spoon the fruit into four small ovenproof dishes. Sprinkle over the mixed/apple pie spice and top with the granola.

3 Bake for 10 minutes until you see the fruit bubbling out the sides. Serve straight away.

Nutrition facts (per serving) Calories 100 Carbohydrate 15g Protein 3g
Fat 3.7g (of which saturates 0.8g)

HERO FOOD: OATS

We've all been told time and time again how porridge/oatmeal is the best start to the day. It is low in fat, high in soluble fibre and is also a great source of complex carbohydrate. This means that it releases energy slowly throughout the day, preventing blood-sugar fluctuations or energy crashes. That said, oats don't necessarily need to be eaten as porridge/oatmeal. You can eat them cold in the form of Bircher's or standard muesli or why not try an Oaty Banana Pancake (see page 195). You could also try Oatcakes (see page 268) or even make your own energy bars to have as a snack pre- or during training. Whichever way, they should definitely be on your list as a go-to food to fuel long endurance training sessions.

Coconut & Mango Rice Pudding

I often recommend rice pudding to my athletes as a recovery choice. The milk content ensures that it has the ideal mix of carbohydrate and protein to repair and recover tired muscles. This recipe is a far cry from the sloppy rice pudding served at school with a dollop of jam!

Serves 4   **Preparation time:** 10 minutes   **Cooking time:** 30 minutes

400ml/14fl oz/generous 1½ cups reduced-fat canned coconut milk
450ml/16fl oz/scant 2 cups skimmed milk
75g/3oz/⅓ cup short-grain pudding rice
55g/2oz/¼ cup caster/granulated sugar
grated zest of 2 limes
juice of 1 lime
1 mango, peeled, pitted and sliced

1 Pour the coconut milk and milk into a saucepan and bring to the boil over a high heat. Turn the heat down to low and add the rice, sugar and lime zest. Simmer gently for about 20 minutes until the rice is soft and has absorbed most of the milk.

2 Meanwhile, drizzle the lime juice over the mango slices and toss together to coat.

3 Spoon the rice pudding into serving bowls and serve hot with the mango slices.

Nutrition facts (per serving) Calories 252 Carbohydrate 50g Protein 5.2g
Fat 5.2g (of which saturates 4.8g)

Baked Spiced Apricots

Full of flavour and valuable nutrients but still good enough to serve at a dinner party! For best results, make sure the apricots are only just ripe.

Serves 4　　**Preparation time:** 5 minutes, plus cooling
Cooking time: 20 minutes

4 tbsp clear honey
3 lime leaves
4 cardamom pods
1 lemongrass stalk
1 tsp grated root ginger
8 apricots

1　Put the honey in a saucepan with 750ml/26fl oz/3 cups water and bring to the boil over a high heat. Turn the heat down to low and simmer gently for a few minutes until the honey has dissolved into the water. Add the lime leaves, cardamom, lemongrass and ginger.

2　Lower the apricots into the saucepan. The syrup mixture should cover them but if it does not, add a little more boiling water. Cover and simmer for about 15 minutes until the apricots are tender. Remove from the heat and leave the apricots in the syrup until cool enough to handle.

3　Take the apricots out of the syrup, cut in half and remove the pits, then divide the apricots among four individual serving dishes.

4　Return the syrup to a high heat and boil for a few minutes until reduced by half. Pour over the apricots and serve hot.

Nutrition facts (per serving)　Calories 97　Carbohydrate 25g　Protein 1g Fat 0g (of which saturates 0g)

Poached Pears with Cardamom Custard

Custard is often overlooked as a dessert these days, but it is an excellent way to ensure you meet your dairy requirements. I have made the custard the main feature in this recipe for that reason and added the poached pears as an accompaniment.

Serves 4   **Preparation time:** 5 minutes   **Cooking time:** 15 minutes

4 ripe pears, peeled, cored and halved
2 tbsp custard powder
500ml/17fl oz/2 cups skimmed milk
1 tbsp caster/granulated sugar
4 cardamom pods

1 Preheat the oven to 150°C/300°F/Gas 2.

2 Put the pear halves in a baking pan with just enough water to cover the base of the pan. Bake for 20 minutes, or until the pears are tender.

3 Meanwhile, make the custard. Put the custard powder in a measuring jug and add 1 tablespoon of the milk to make a paste. Put the rest of the milk, the sugar and cardamom pods in a saucepan and bring to the boil over a high heat.

4 Pour the milk mixture onto the custard paste in the measuring jug, whisking continuously so they blend completely without forming any lumps. Pour the contents of the jug back into the saucepan, turn the heat down to low and cook for about 5 minutes, stirring continuously, until the custard is thick.

5 Pour the custard over the pears and serve hot.

Nutrition facts (per serving) Calories 215 Carbohydrate 50g Protein 5g
Fat 0g (of which saturates 0g)

GLOSSARY

acetyl co-enzyme A (acetyl-CoA) is an important molecule in metabolism, used in many biochemical reactions.

adenosine triphosphate (ATP) is a molecule that transports chemical energy within cells for metabolism.

adipose tissue is the scientific term for fat stores.

aerobic metabolism involves the production of energy via biochemical pathways in the presence of oxygen.

alpha-linolenic acid (ALA) is an essential omega-3 fatty acid necessary for growth and development.

amino acids – protein plays a crucial role in almost all biological processes and amino acids are the building blocks of it. Branched-chain amino acids are essential nutrients that the body obtains from proteins found in food – especially meat, dairy products and legumes. They include leucine, isoleucine and valine. 'Branched-chain' refers to the chemical structure of these amino acids.

anaerobic metabolism involves the production of energy via biochemical pathways in the absence of oxygen.

antioxidants are enzymes or other organic substances, such as vitamin E or beta-carotene, capable of counteracting the damaging effects of oxidation in animal tissues.

autoimmune condition – your body's immune system protects you from disease and infection. But if you have an autoimmune disease, your immune system attacks healthy cells in your body by mistake. Autoimmune diseases can affect many parts of the body.

beta-alanine is a naturally occurring amino acid used in athletes to help reduce acid levels when exercising at high intensity.

bioelectrical impedance testing is a commonly used method for estimating body composition, and in particular body fat.

body composition is the term used to measure levels of fat mass and non-fat mass. It is often expressed as body fat percentage.

Borg Scale – the recognized scale for measuring the level of exertion.

BW stands for body weight. In sports nutrition, calculations are worked out per kg of body weight.

cardiovascular system is an organ system that circulates blood, transporting nutrients, oxygen, carbon dioxide, hormones and blood cells to and from cells in the body to nourish it and help to fight diseases, stabilize body temperature and pH, and to maintain homeostasis.

co-enzymes are organic molecules that are required by certain enzymes to carry out reactions.

co-factors are often classified as inorganic substances that are required for, or increase the rate of, reactions.

creatine phosphate (CP) is a molecule that provides a rapidly transferable reserve of high energy into muscles and the brain.

curcumin is the principle component of the spice turmeric and a powerful antioxidant.

delayed onset muscle soreness (DOMS) is the pain and stiffness felt in muscles several hours to days after unaccustomed or strenuous exercise.

DHA, or docosahexaenoic acid, is an omega-3 fatty acid that is a primary structural component of the human brain.

electrolytes refers to salts such as sodium, potassium, magnesium etc. that are needed by the working muscle during exercise. Sodium and potassium help to draw water in and prevent dehydration, while magnesium is necessary for muscle contraction.

enzymes are biological macro molecules that are responsible for thousands of metabolic processes that sustain life.

EPA, or eicosapentaenoic acid, is an omega-3 fatty acid found in fish oils and shown to help reduce inflammation and reduce cholesterol levels.

ergogenic aids are any external substances, such as caffeine, that can be determined to enhance performance in high-intensity exercises.

fatty acids make up the acid part of a fat molecule and can be either saturated or unsaturated.

fasted state when you have not eaten for a period of more than 6 hours.

fast-twitch muscle fibres are good for rapid movements like jumping to catch a ball or sprinting for the bus. They contract quickly, but get tired fast, as they consume lots of energy.

fat adapted – a method of eating and training that helps to improve the efficiency of using fat as fuel for endurance events.

follicular phase refers to the time of your menstrual cycle leading up to ovulation.

free radicals are atoms or groups of atoms and can be formed when oxygen interacts with certain molecules. Once formed, these highly reactive radicals can start a chain reaction, like dominoes. Their chief danger comes from the damage they can do when they react with important cellular components such as DNA, or the cell membrane.

GI (glycaemic index) is a rating system for foods containing carbohydrates. It shows how quickly each food affects your blood sugar (glucose) level when that food is eaten on its own.

glycogen is the body's store of glucose in muscles and liver when glucose is not needed at that moment in time. Glycogen is readily converted to glucose and transported to the working muscles on demand by the body.

glycolysis is the breakdown of glucose by enzymes into pyruvic and lactic acids, releasing energy in the absence of oxygen.

gluconeogenesis is the breakdown of non carbohydrate substrates such as fatty acids (fats) and amino acids (protein) to produce glucose for energy when there is not sufficient carbohydrate available.

glucose is a simple sugar and the principle source of energy for all living organisms.

gluten – protein found in wheat responsible for giving wheat dough its elastic nature.

haemoglobin is the iron-containing oxygen-transport protein in the red blood cells. Haemoglobin in the blood carries oxygen from the respiratory organs (lungs or gills) to the rest of the body (i.e. the tissues).

isoflavanoids are a classification of anti-oxidants.

lactate – a waste product of anaerobic respiration that accumulates in muscles during exercise.

lactate threshold – the point at which the levels of lactate in the blood are too high to be cleared by the oxygen available during exercise.

luteal phase is the period of time in the menstrual cycle post ovulation.

macronutrients are energy-providing chemical substances consumed by organisms in large quantities. The three macronutrients in nutrition are carbohydrates, lipids and proteins.

metabolic rate refers to the rate of energy expenditure.

micronutrients are nutrients required by humans and other organisms throughout life in small quantities.

mitochondria are the 'powerhouse of the cell' because they generate most of the cell's supply of adenosine triphosphate (ATP).

mmol (millimole) a unit of measurement equivalent to 1/1000 of a mole where a mole is 1 molecule.

motor control is the process by which humans and animals use their neuromuscular system to activate and co-ordinate the muscles and limbs involved in the performance of a motor skill.

muscle contraction refers to the shortening or tensing of muscle fibres.

muscle hypertrophy refers to increasing the size of muscle fibres within a muscle.

muscle mass is the term used when talking about the amount of muscle within a body.

muscle protein synthesis is the building of muscle.

myocytes are the structural cells of a muscle.

myofibrils are the contractile fibre within muscle.

neuro-muscular system is the collective term for the muscles of the body, together with the nerves supplying them.

osteoporosis is a disorder in which the bones become increasingly porous, brittle and subject to fracture, owing to loss of calcium and other mineral components.

oxidative stress is damage to cell membranes within the body caused by free radicals.

phytates are a component of some high-fibre foods, including many cereal grains, which may, in excessive amounts, cause constipation or interfere with the body's ability to absorb minerals.

plyometrics is a system of dynamic muscle exercise, designed to develop power for running, jumping and throwing sports. It is based on the principle that muscles contract faster and with greater force when worked from a pre-stretched position.

polyphenols are organic compounds responsible for the colour and flavour of some fruits and vegetables; they may have antioxidant properties.

protein pulsing is the term used in sports nutrition when describing consumption of 0.25g/kg BW protein at regular intervals through the day to maximize muscle protein synthesis.

pyruvate is the end product of glycolysis and may be metabolized to lactate or to acetyl CoA.

rate of perceived exertion (RPE) is a scale used to measure the intensity of exercise. The RPE scale runs from 0–10 where 0 is being still and 10 is maximal intensity.

resynthesize is when depleted stores such as glycogen are rebuilt post exercise.

turbo session is a high-intensity bike session done indoors. The bike is attached to a platform so that it stays stationary while the individual can complete a workout.

BIBLIOGRAPHY

http://www.anorexiabulimiacare.org.uk/

Burke, Louise, *Clinical Sports Nutrition*, 4th edition, 2010, McGraw-Hill Medical Publishing

Burke, Louise, *Practical Sports Nutrition*, 2007, Human Kinetics Publishing

Burke, Louise, et al., 'Nutrition for athletes, a position paper by nutrition working group of the IOC, International Olympic Committee', 2012

Drobinic, F., et al., 'Reduction of delayed onset muscle soreness by a novel curcumin delivery system (Meriva®): a randomised, placebo-controlled trial', *Journal of the International Society of Sports Nutrition*, June 18, 2014

Eddy, Kate, *Strength and Conditioning*, colleague's notes – unpublished, 2014

Fuhrman, Dr Joel, et al., 'Fuelling the vegetarian (vegan) athlete', *Current Sports Medicine: Reports*, 2010, Vol. 9, No. 4

Gluek, C. J., et al., 'Severe vitamin D deficiency, myopathy and rhabdomyolysis', *North American Journal of Medical Sciences*, August 2013, volume 5, issue 8

Hausswirth, Christophe, et al., 'Physiological and nutritional aspects of post-exercise recovery specific recommendations for female athletes', *Sports Medicine Journal*, 2011; 41 (10): 861–882

Helms, Eric R., et al., 'A systematic review of dietary protein during caloric restriction in resistance trained lean athletes: A case for higher intakes', *International Journal of Sport Nutrition and Exercise*, 2014 Apr; 24(2): 127–38

Isacco, L., et al., 'Influence of hormonal status on substrate utilization at rest and during exercise in the female population', *Sports Medicine Journal*: 2012 Apr 1;42(4):327–42

Jeukendrup, Asker, 'A step towards personalized sports nutrition: carbohydrate intake during exercise', *Sports Medicine Journal* (2014) 44 (Suppl 1): S25–S33

Kerksick, Chad et al., 'International Society of Sports Nutrition position stand: Nutrient timing', *Journal of the International Society of Sports Nutrition*, 2008 Oct 3

Łagowska, K., et al., 'Effects of dietary intervention in young female athletes with menstrual disorders', *Journal of the International Society of Sports Nutrition* (2014) 11:21

Lenn, J. et al., 'The effects of fish oil and isoflavones on delayed onset muscle soreness', *Medical Science, Sports and Exercise*, 2002 Oct; 34(10):1605–13

Oosthuyse, T., et al., 'The effect of the menstrual cycle on exercise metabolism: implications for exercise performance in eumenorrhoeic women', *Sports Medicine Journal*, 2010 Mar 1;40(3): 207–27

Phillips, Stuart M., 'Dietary protein requirements and adaptive advantages in athletes', *British Journal of Nutrition* (2012), 108, S158–S167

Phillips, Stuart M., 'Protein consumption and resistance exercise: maximizing anabolic potential', *Sports Science Exchange* (2013) Vol. 26, No. 107, 1–5

Phillips, Stuart M., et al., 'The role of milk- and soy-based protein in support of muscle protein synthesis and muscle protein accretion in young and elderly persons', *Journal of the American College of Nutrition* (2009) Vol. 28, No. 4, 343–354

Spriet, Lawrence L., 'New insights into the interaction of carbohydrate and fat metabolism during exercise', *Sports Medicine Journal* (2014) 44 (Suppl 1): S87–S96

Stark, Matthew, et al., 'Protein timing and its effects on muscular hypertrophy and strength in individuals engaged in weight-training', *Journal of the International Society of Sports Nutrition*, 2012, 9:54

Wardle, Katie RD, et al., 'The nutritional demands of ultra-endurance running', www.ultrarunningltd.co.uk/training-schedule/nutrition/nutritional-demands-of-ultra-running

Williams, N.I., et al., 'Evidence for a causal role of low energy availability in the induction of menstrual cycle disturbances during strenuous exercise training', *The Journal of Clinical Endocrinology & Metabolism*, 2001: 86:5184–93

Wilmore, J.H. and Costill, D.L., *Physiology of Sport and Exercise*, 3rd edition, 2005, Human Kinetics Publishing

INDEX

ACKNOWLEDGMENTS

There are many people I would like to thank for helping me to produce this book.

I must thank Nourish Books for their support from start to finish, but special thanks to Rebecca Woods and Judy Barratt, without whom I think I would have given up on many occasions!

I also need to pay a special thanks to Kate Eddy, a dear friend but also one of the best strength and conditioning coaches I have had the privilege to work with. She has helped me to have a better understanding of the importance of strength and conditioning. Together we have worked with many athletes, resulting in successful outcomes. Without her guidance and expertise the section on strength and conditioning would not have been possible.

I want to pay special thanks to my friends and family – Mum, Dad and my sister – who have supported and encouraged me all the way through this experience, and to Holly Rush for writing the foreword and being a constant source of inspiration.

Special thanks also to all the athletes I have worked with over the years, as you have helped shaped this book. There are too many of you to name individually, but you all know who you are!

A final thanks to my extremely supportive husband, two beautiful daughters and crazy spaniel. Andrew you have kept me grounded throughout this writing adventure; Maya and Ella you just make me proud everyday and now I hope I have returned this back to you. And Bailey, without our long trail runs together I'm not sure I would have come up with so many ideas on how to write this book!